Champion's Story

Jonathan Powell is the Racing Editor of the *Sunday People* and has been a close friend of Bob Champion for many years. He is also the author of *Monksfield* (1980).

D0544699

Bob Champion *and* Jonathan Powell

CHAMPION'S STORY

A Great Human Triumph

FONTANA PAPERBACKS

First published by Victor Gollancz Ltd 1981
First issued in Fontana Paperbacks 1982
Second impression February 1984

Copyright © Bob Champion & Jonathan Powell 1981

Made and printed in Great Britain
by William Collins Sons & Co. Ltd, Glasgow

Dedication

I would like to dedicate this book to all the people who gave me hope when there was precious little else to cling to, in particular my parents, my sister Mary, her husband Richard and their two children Nicky and Emma; the doctors, nurses and staff of the Royal Marsden Hospital; Josh Gifford and his team of owners; Burly Cocks—and, of course, Aldaniti.

Bob Champion

Acknowledgements

This book could not have been completed without the kindness and encouragement of those closest to Bob Champion during his long illness and recovery. In particular I would like to thank Richard and Mary Hussey, who were unfailingly helpful; Josh and Althea Gifford who, typically, played down their vital role in this story. Carol and Jenny, two of the nurses from the Pinkham ward, provided invaluable assistance and helped to clarify and check the considerable medical detail; and the guidance and support of Dr Jane Merrow, too, was much appreciated.

I would also like to thank Colm Farren and Pip Pocock for their generous assistance, and the lovely Sarah Reeves for transforming the original manuscript into immaculate order.

For reasons of medical ethics the name of Bob's doctor has been changed to Dr Jane Merrow.

Jonathan Powell
May 1981

List of Illustrations

Chapter 1

BOB CHAMPION LOOKED remarkably healthy for a man who had just been given eight months to live. Eight lingering, distressing, increasingly painful months unless he agreed immediately to a drastic new type of treatment which promised, but could not guarantee, a complete recovery. Rays of sunshine glinting through the window of the small hospital consulting room lit up the impressive bronze tan on his worried features. Young, fit, successful, at the very pinnacle of his eventful career, he listened in disbelief as two doctors explained again their shattering verdict that he had cancer in two parts of his body.

The news that his very life was threatened by the most dreaded and vicious of modern diseases was shocking enough, but he found it even harder to comprehend because he had never felt so well. A fearless, tough and resourceful steeplechase jockey, aged thirty-one, he had won upwards of 350 races in the previous twelve years. Now that part of his life was ended—perhaps permanently—by something over which he had no control at all. After a summer's holiday in America he had returned home, mildly anxious about an irritating lump on one of his testicles. Despite two subsequent painful exploratory operations he still had not come to terms with the fact that he had cancer.

Jump racing, by its very nature, is a hazardous business. When you are riding for a fall the risks can be appallingly high. Jockeys accept the brutal fact that it's a question of when rather than if they will be seriously hurt. Theirs is such a dangerous occupation that a series of insurance and compensation schemes provided for them have proved woefully inadequate. So Bob Champion was used to waking up to the unique smell and discomfort of hospital life. Breaks, cracks, bruises and concussion from falls he understood

11

only too well. Cancer, that most treacherous of diseases, was altogether more frightening. How could he begin to face something he could not see, let alone feel? During the first ten minutes of the interview with two specialists he barely heard a word in the hospital room early in August, 1979. Waves of panic surged through his body and for the first time, he admitted later, he was petrified. What had he done to deserve such an unkind fate?

Bob tried to concentrate as the male doctor continued to speak; he listened incredulously as it was explained again that the first operation, almost three weeks earlier, to remove one of his testicles, had established that an uncomfortable lump there had been a malignant tumour. After an endless series of tests, X-rays and body scans, a second operation, which involved the removal of part of a rib, had confirmed the doctors' fears that the cancer from the tumour had spread into the lymph glands in his chest. The choice, the doctor explained, was straightforward. Bob could start, at once, revolutionary chemotherapy treatment that offered a solid chance of saving his life. Or he would die.

"How long have I left?" Bob asked quietly.

"It could be as little as eight months," replied the doctor. "Perhaps two or three months more."

"If I don't have the treatment will I be able to go on riding for a while?" he queried, desperately seeking an escape route from the implications of the doctors' grim diagnosis.

"For a few months perhaps."

"What about radiation?"

Radiation alone, the doctors explained gravely, could not possibly cope with the swift spread of cancer in his body. His particular type of cancer was already far advanced at stage three. Until the early seventies, they added significantly, there had been no effective cure.

"Is there no other way?"

"No, I'm afraid not."

"Then I'll take my chance and continue riding," Bob said stubbornly. "If I'm to die I'd rather it happens while I'm doing something I love rather than lying wasting away in a hospital bed."

The two doctors exchanged glances. Argument, let alone resistance, was not a reaction they usually encountered in similar circumstances. After an awkward silence the second doctor, Jane Merrow, again painstakingly explained the effects and results of the new chemotherapy treatment that he must agree to undergo.

The system, perfected in America, had produced an excellent percentage of fully cured patients . . . but he must be prepared to face the most dire side effects caused by the powerful dosage of drugs. Bob would be violently sick, lose all his hair and suffer agonizing constipation. He would, in addition, succumb to the slimmer's disease anorexia and almost certainly would become sterile and thus be unable to have children. He would need a minimum of four cycles of chemotherapy treatment to have any chance of a complete cure. Each cycle would last twenty-one days of which he had to spend six in hospital while the drugs that would save his life were administered intravenously. During the remaining fifteen days he would need to be nursed constantly as he would be far too ill, most of the time, to fend for himself. His riding career would have to be postponed for many months—and was quite possibly ended—but he had an excellent chance of a complete recovery.

Still Bob Champion resisted the pressure to agree to have the treatment. He could not afford a year's absence in such a competitive sport. His chief employer, the brilliant young trainer Josh Gifford, however sympathetic, would surely have to engage another experienced jockey in his absence and Bob himself would soon be forgotten.

Dr Jane Merrow remembers that day. "I put it to Bob that it would be the height of folly to have only approximately one more year to live when he could have the rest of his life if he consented to have the treatment. The argument took a surprisingly long time considering he really did not have a choice. I don't think anyone in his position takes that sort of thing in first time, all at once. He was having to adjust to the idea of everything in his life having to stop at once at that point. He was much more obsessed initially with his lost rides than with the treatment itself. . . .

"No-one to my knowledge has ever turned down the treatment but at first Bob was very determined that he would go on riding regardless. He was extremely stubborn, quite bolshie about it really. He was more articulate than most people we treat. Few patients argue back. He was more insistent than most, because, presumably, he had more to lose than most," she says.

Still the argument persisted. Bob explains:

Well, how would you feel? I'd heard quite a lot about cancer but had never given it a second thought. Cancer, to me, was the same sort of thing as bad car accidents. Something that happened to other people.

Finally Bob's knowledge of betting and odds proved decisive. "What are my chances exactly?" he asked.

"If you start the chemotherapy immediately you have a seventy-five per cent chance of a full recovery," replied Dr Merrow.

Bob still remembers vividly his feeling of relief when he heard that precise percentage.

When you are in racing you understand odds and those sounded pretty hopeful to me. Her statistics persuaded me to go ahead and take her advice. If the odds had been seventy per cent or below there was no way I was going to have the treatment.

You see, despite everything the two doctors had told me and the two operations, I could not accept I was seriously ill because I had never felt so fit and well. Never. They told me later that feeling so well was another symptom of my type of cancer. So many things upset me that day but worst of all was the thought of not being able to have my own children. That was a cruel blow and one I still haven't come to terms with.

The other thing that hit me hard was the prospect of losing all my hair. Dr Merrow had already told me I was going to feel bloody awful and now she was saying I would look bloody awful too. I hated the thought of going bald and so tried to believe it wouldn't happen.

One more crucial doubt remained. Would he be able to ride again when the treatment was completed?

Dr Merrow had no experience of treating a professional sportsman for Bob's type of cancer but she concedes, "I didn't really think he would return to riding again. No, I didn't. His was a very serious illness and I knew how damaging the side effects of the drugs would be, especially on his lungs. In many walks of life if you are out of action for at all long, then the chances are that you don't get back. I knew nothing of racing but imagined the same rule applied. Bob asked me if I thought he would be able to ride again and I must have said it would depend on how he responded to the treatment, that I could not see any reason why not if he came through it well enough. But privately I had my doubts."

The decision was taken that Bob Champion would begin his first course that very day. He sat, unhearing, as if in a trance as the two doctors outlined the various tests he must take that morning. His brain, numb with shock, refused to take in any more medical details and his mind drifted back over his riding career to his early life with his family in Yorkshire.

Chapter 2

WHEN BOB CHAMPION was born on 4th June 1948 he seemed destined to a life on horseback pursuing foxes across the English countryside. No less than seven generations of his family have been professional huntsmen. His father, Bob senior, a fearless, accomplished horseman, certainly expected him to follow in his hoofbeats, but mutters sadly, "As a small boy our Bob was not keen on horses at all. All he wanted to do was go down to the nearby farm and drive the tractors." His son's initial dislike of horses may be explained by a painful and frightening incident when he was barely old enough to walk. His father persuaded him to try to jump his pony over a ladder and he fell off into a bed of stinging nettles.

Bob's mother Phyllis, quiet and undemonstrative, comes from a farming family. His father, a forceful character, is a tough ex-soldier who nearly lost an arm in the battle for Arnhem. All the nerves in his right hand were shot away, and he was in and out of hospital for twelve months. Skilful surgery saved the arm from being amputated though he was left with a permanent lack of feeling and strength, but even so he was eventually able to resume his first love, hunting, at first in Kent and later in the North of England with the Cleveland pack of foxhounds run by the genial old Master, Major Leslie Petch. He remained with the Cleveland for seventeen years. Other members of young Bob's family maintain the Champion links with hunting: Uncle Jack is with the Old Surrey Hounds, Uncle Nimrod is with the Ledbury Foxhounds and his cousin Bridger also worked for a while with the Croome pack.

After his initial disaster on horseback Bob preferred walking hounds at exercise for mile after mile, helping out on the local farm, fishing and going off with his father to distant farms to collect dead meat for the hounds. " 'Knackerin', we called it," says his father. At the age of nine Bob was ready to try riding again. He would disappear from the house, pop into the stable yard, saddle his pony and go off on his own. Gradually, as they hacked around the fields, his confidence grew. Then with the gentle support of a family friend, Margaret Silman, he started hunting. When they reached a jump she would cross it on her own horse, tether it up, clamber back across the obstacle, climb on Bob's pony and jump that over too. Bob, meanwhile, would scramble through the hedge as best he could on his own two legs.

Margaret Silman encouraged Bob to ride as much as possible and a farmer's son, David Anker, who had recently joined the Cleveland Hunt as whipper-in, took Bob under his protective wing. Bob, by now aged ten, was still a little apprehensive about falling off until the day a girlfriend at school asked him to help start her pony jumping. With a gallantry that was to win many a girl's heart in future years he readily agreed to her request. He says:

> This particular pony would not jump anything with the girl on it so I decided it was time to sort it out. I was a bit nervous at first but showing off in front of her gave me sufficient courage and so I followed David Anker straight over a five-barred gate. The pony jumped it well, I stayed on and was so pleased with myself I turned round and jumped the gate twice more. After that you couldn't stop me from trying to jump anything. I was crazy about riding.

His sister Mary, eighteen months younger and much smaller, was also a natural and fearless rider. Bob and Mary had a volatile relationship which still exists today. They would fight like cat and dog but would unite if anyone criticized either of them. When their parents were out Bob's favourite pastime was to bully Mary. He would find a sixpence, throw it into the nearest field, then seize a hunting crop and say, "Right, on your knees and find the sixpence." If Mary stood up before she found the coin he would give her a crack with the whip. "He was an evil little horror!" Mary exclaims—and no wonder.

Once, on a chilly winter's afternoon, Bob and Mary set off for tea with their friends the Thompsons. Bored with standing at the bus stop they starting fighting, and by the time the bus arrived the pair were locked in muddy combat at the bottom of a ditch. After waiting patiently for a while the bus driver left the two Champions still battling away furiously in the ditch. They were aged eleven and nine.

"Nothing frightened Bob even at that age," Bob Champion senior says proudly. "Once he came home from school with a black eye. A friend of mine told me later that Bob had sorted out three bullies at school though he never mentioned it. He was a quiet lad, liked to be on his own, though sometimes as a treat we would let him go with the kennelmen to Middlesbrough to watch the wrestling."

Even as a small boy Bob showed unusual determination. When only twelve he was the youngest finisher from his school in the testing Lykewake Walk—a forty-mile hike across the Yorkshire moors. "When he returned home his feet were badly swollen," his mother recalls, "but he had been too stubborn to give up. He came in late on Sunday morning, ate a little lunch then slept for over twenty-four hours."

Bob's closest friends, then and now, were Derek and Howard Thompson, sons of a local businessman who lived at Nunthorpe. The Thompsons remain his adopted family. The trio would go hunting and racing together and became involved in the usual boyish scrapes. They would attend Redcar races with Bob's father whose duty was to take the knacker van there in case any horses were killed. The parking spot for the van was opposite the winning post and grandstand. On the other side of the course stood the television commentary box, usually occupied by ITV's immaculate, carnationed, hat-raising front-man John Rickman—and now, twenty years later, frequently inhabited by Bob's childhood friend, that same Derek Thompson.

One day at a televised Redcar meeting an expected interviewee failed to turn up. Rickman, desperate for someone to interrogate, urgently grabbed the three small boys lurking close to his position. After the usual banal chatter John asked each of the boys what they planned to be when they grew up. Bob and Howard replied that they wanted to be jockeys and Derek said he would like to be a BBC commentator. Only Howard failed to fulfil those heady ambitions though, as his brother confirms, he was the best rider of all at the time and subsequently won a few point-to-points—races for horses that hunt regularly through the winter.

Bob's desire to become a jockey was strengthened the day he and two other lads were asked to round up loose horses during the afternoon at the Cleveland Hunt point-to-point. Major Petch, who ran the meeting with his usual military precision, was so pleased with their efforts that after the last race he allowed them to hold their own private race. Bob won easily on a retired racehorse, Apple Tea, and from that moment was more determined than ever to be a jockey. Major Petch, however, was less pleased with Bob and Derek when they tried to round up a herd of sheep in the middle of a hunt on Lord Guisborough's estate near Tocketts. Inspired by a film they had seen starring John Wayne, they charged across the field, scattering horses and hounds. The sheep stampeded, burst through a fence and disappeared in all directions. The boys' punishment was to be banned from the hunting field for several weeks.

Bob viewed his school merely as a nuisance which interfered with his hunting arrangements. He showed little inclination for book-work, read only comics, but developed a considerable aptitude for engineering, woodwork and metalwork. Team games did not appeal at all, though he revealed unexpected skills at pole vaulting.

"Although Bob was useless at cricket," Derek Thompson remembers, "we drafted him in at the last minute one day as a wicket keeper. Someone threw the ball in to Bob, he missed it and the ball bounced off his head. The blow put a dent in the ball but didn't seem to affect Bob at all. In those days he was a quiet lad, very shy, but he had a killer streak in him and a hell of a temper on occasions. He was a brilliant mechanic, very clever with his hands, a perfectionist at anything he attempted."

As soon as Bob was fifteen the decision was taken to send him south to Wiltshire where he could live and work on a farm owned by his uncle Arthur Corp, and could also attend the technical college a few miles away at Trowbridge. Arthur and Eileen Corp farmed over three hundred acres but the attraction for their young nephew was that they always kept at least one point-to-point horse in training each season.

Bob started working for them in the autumn of 1963 on the

princely wage of one pound a week. The routine was hard and tiring for a boy fresh from school. He would be out in the farmyard soon after six, muck out the boxes of two or three horses, saddle one of them, and exercise it on the farm for an hour or so. Then he would snatch a bite of breakfast and catch the bus into Trowbridge seven miles away. A second bus took him to the gates of the college where he was studying for an engineering diploma. In the evening he would return to the farm, dress over the horses, feed them and do other odd jobs before supper. At weekends in the winter he was able to go hunting on Saturdays.

Arthur Corp admits grudgingly in cidery tones, "Ah, if he'd stayed at the job he would have made a proper farmer. He was very good at tractor driving, ploughing, cultivating and such like—but he was a waste of time when I put him to hoeing between the mangles. He and the cows did not seem to get on either, but he was a natural when it came to race riding."

The point-to-point season began, as usual, in February. Bob had a dozen rides spread over four months but his first, on his uncle's Holmcourt, was a disaster.

> I came to the last fence with a bit of a chance but my horse fell. I remember hitting the ground very, very hard, picking myself up, counting the bruises and thinking this game is not for me.

In March Bob rode his first winner, on Holmcourt, a small, eleven-year-old mare, in the Tedworth Adjacent Hunts race at Larkhill. Next time out he fell with Holmcourt again, but in April he won his second race on her in the Craven Farmers race at Lockinge on the same day his cousin, Billy Champion, won the Open on Domaboy. Bob was fifteen years old and already knew what he was going to do with his life.

> By now I was certain I was going to be a jockey. My father had been great friends all his life with Jim Fairgrieve, head lad to the best jumping trainer in the country, Peter Cazalet. My sister used to go down to his stables in Kent and ride out for a few weeks each summer and I always tried to fit in the odd weekend there. I was fascinated by such a well organized racing set up and was

keen to join it but Jim thought I was too heavy to start as a professional and advised riding as an amateur at first to get more opportunities.

Bob left Trowbridge College after a year with an engineering diploma and spent the next three years working for his uncle on the farm at an increased wage of five pounds a week. More point-to-point rides came his way. The best horse he rode was Gipsy Melody, a brilliant prospect owned by his uncle. Gipsy Melody won twice as a six-year-old in 1965 but for the rest of her racing career respiratory problems prevented her fulfilling her immense promise. Bob remembers her with affection.

She was just about the best jumper I've ridden all through the years, a brilliant athlete and she used to gain so much ground at the obstacles. I suppose I was too brave in those days but at the time she seemed the ideal partner; yet often when I asked her to quicken at the end of a race she would gurgle as if she couldn't get her breath.

"They were a right combination," Arthur Corp says, "but in later years Gipsy Melody ran even better for Bob's sister Mary who won quite a few races on her. Now *she could* ride. In all the time Bob was with me he only lost one race he should have won, at Larkhill against a top class hunter-chaser, Lizzy the Lizzard, ridden by a very clever and experienced jockey, David Maundrell.

"Bob told me before the race he was determined to jump the last fence beside David Maundrell on Lizzy the Lizzard and then out-ride him on the run to the winning post. I told him not to leave it as late as that but he was a stubborn boy and wouldn't listen. Sure enough, Bob tried to be too smart. The two horses were in the air together at the last fence but David Maundrell and Lizzy the Lizzard were a bit too strong for them on the run-in. Bob came back in a terrible temper but I'm sure he learned a valuable lesson that day."

One man suitably impressed with Bob's skill as a horseman was Peter Calver, a big, genial man who somehow reduced his large frame sufficiently each spring to ride in point-to-points. Calver, a local vet, farmer and trainer, had discovered the future Grand National winner Highland Wedding two years previously and had won several races on the horse before selling him on to his close friend Toby Balding. Calver urged Bob to consider becoming a jockey:

"I told Bob there was a job for him any time he wanted with Toby Balding and that in my opinion he would be mad to turn down such a good chance. He didn't need much persuading. There was a devious motive to my good deed. Bob was far too good for point-to-points and kept pinching my rides so that was the best way I could think of getting rid of him!"

So in August 1967, Bob joined Toby Balding's team at Fyfield, near Andover in Hampshire, as one of several amateur jockeys in the stable. He was also given a vague role as farm manager to justify his amateur status.

Eileen Corp recalls: "His heart was set on becoming a jockey and we didn't have nearly enough horses to keep him happy. Anyway our home was becoming a bit quiet for him. For the first two years he didn't go out at all but then he went wild. He had a different girlfriend every time he was out yet thought so little of them he couldn't remember most of their names. He was a devil."

Toby Balding, a big, untidy, bespectacled figure, was and is a trainer who tends to have almost as many jockeys in his stable as horses. Even so Bob was promised race rides at once since Toby has always seen the benefit of using the claiming allowance of inexperienced jockeys to reduce the weight on his horses.

Bob's introduction to a professional racing stable could not have been more disastrous. On his second morning at the yard he was legged aboard Dozo, a useful handicap chaser who had only just come back into training after a summer spent out at grass. As Bob landed on his back Dozo, unused to such a weighty imposition, reared over backwards, pinning his rider to the ground. As his ankle hit the concrete Bob heard the crack of broken bones. He had broken his left ankle and several bones in his foot. When he was taken to Odstock Hospital near Salisbury, the ankle started to swell up so massively that doctors decided to wait a few days before operating. A week later the broken bones were pinned and the leg put in plaster. The pin is still there today. The anaesthetist during the operation was a remarkable woman, Mrs Mita Easton who breeds, rides and trains her own horses. During the next few days she became firm friends with Bob and later was to provide him with several winners on her horses. A delightful eccentric, Mrs Easton, now in her mid-sixties, has recently retired from Odstock Hospital but still trains her horses and runs her own pub, the Sheaf of Arrows, at Cranborne in Dorset. She had never ridden until she was left a horse in a will in 1945. Later she started riding in point-to-points.

"Did you win a race?" I inquired.

"Oh, no, not at all! I never even once got round. But I was picked up by some very nice people when I fell off," she replied. "Bob was always a lovely horseman, he had the most superb hands but I formed the impression he didn't like me ringing him up at five in the morning to book him to ride my horses."

When Bob was allowed out of hospital he worked in Toby Balding's office until the injury mended. His job as farm manager seemed forgotten. Toby Balding gave Bob his first chance on a modest novice, Swiss Knight, over fences at Worcester at the end of October. Swiss Knight was so far behind after a mile that Bob pulled him up. Next time at Fontwell Swiss Knight started at 66-1 in a seven-horse race and much to his young jockey's surprise, they finished third. Toby Balding trained another novice chaser, Altercation, which was considered even more useless than Swiss Knight. Altercation had fallen on his first run over hurdles two years previously and had fallen consistently over the larger fences in steeplechases. He had yet to finish a race. Toby Balding, in his wisdom, decided to run both horses over fences in the same race at Plumpton in November.

Clive Bailey, who rode Altercation, takes up the story: "Neither of us had a prayer of winning so just for fun Bob and I had a side bet to see who would last the furthest. Bob's horse was a bit free early on and shot off out of control but after a circuit he began to drop back and, to my surprise, my horse started to run. As soon as I passed him I started laughing like hell and then mine turned a somersault at the next fence. As I lay groaning in the mud Bob came by grinning from ear to ear, and pulled up after struggling over one more fence."

On 21st November Bob finished second at Fontwell on the useful mare Last Town, owned and trained by Mrs Easton, but four days later racing came to an abrupt and unscheduled halt. The foot and mouth epidemic sweeping the country causing the slaughter of millions of farm animals had reached such alarming proportions that the Jockey Club took the unprecedented step of closing down racing from 25th November to 5th January. It was a miserable time for everyone in racing. Bob Champion, pleased that his ankle had mended so well, waited impatiently for the ban to end. Racing resumed, briefly, on 5th January but after two days bad weather closed things down for another ten days.

Bob's first ride when the weather cleared was on the dangerous Altercation at Plumpton in yet another novice chase.

The horse started at 20-1 but anyone looking at his record would not have backed him at 200-1. He was hardly the ideal ride for someone as inexperienced as me but in those days I was so keen I would have ridden anything provided its eyesight was all right. If you want to get started as a jump jockey you have to ride the wild and dangerous horses, the ones that the older and wiser jockeys reject as what we call death machines.

Well, everyone in the yard laid bets on how far I would survive and I was sure the horse would bury me. We were all wrong. He jumped well throughout, led three fences out and won nicely. I couldn't believe my luck. I thought I was Lester Piggott and even Toby was pleased.

The celebrations did not last long. Altercation, again ridden by Bob Champion, returned to Plumpton a fortnight later, bulldozed several of the fences as if they were his personal enemy and finally fell heavily at the ninth fence. Bob was knocked out and woke up in the ambulance room with concussion and cuts on his head that required several stitches at the local hospital. Later in the evening he discharged himself but he did not return to Fyfield until six o'clock the next morning. That was the first time he had suffered concussion and he still claims, quite seriously, that he cannot remember where he spent the intervening hours.

Bob rode several winners in the next few months including Last Town for Mrs Easton at Lingfield. On her previous run Last Town had finished second to the subsequent Grand National winner Gay Trip; and thirteen years later Last Town's son Martinstown was a fancied runner in the 1981 Grand National.

Bob shared a house at Fyfield with a clutch of hopeful young jockeys including Clive Bailey, Christy Mellerick, Martin Blackshaw, Jim Old and Gardie Grissell. All six rode winners for the stable and Martin, Jim and Gardie are now successful trainers.

In between injuries Bob was an occasional member of Toby Balding's Sunday football team. By no means a natural ball player he was chosen at left back alongside the large, bespectacled, solid and ungainly figure of the trainer. Bob's burgeoning football career was brought to an abrupt and painful conclusion by yet another injury inflicted this time by his own captain, the team's destroyer Toby Balding. Bob was perhaps a little slow to clear a cross, the opposing centre forward was about to shoot, so Balding, in desperation, launched a typically scything tackle, kicked Bob and the ball, putting them both out of the game. Bob was carried off in agony with damaged ankle ligaments. The ankle came up like a balloon and he was unable to ride for three weeks. Toby Balding, I regret to report, is still sometimes loosed on unsuspecting opponents on the football field.

Bob's was not the only unusual soccer accident at Fyfield. Clement Freud, one of the stable's owners and now a member of Parliament, ended the active career of Tommy Docherty in friendly and charity games. Docherty, once the hard man of Scottish football, was by then a club manager. Freud was so incensed by the Doc's unnecessarily crude tackle on Toby's brother Ian that he ran fully thirty yards across the field before delivering his own rather unorthodox challenge. The impact of the two men sent Docherty limping off the field never to return. At least on this occasion the pair were on opposite sides.

Toby Balding was, and is, a warm, friendly, fun-loving man who treats his racing team as a large, happy family. This good-natured attitude has never prevented him, however, from bawling out his jockeys and lads in the strongest possible language when he feels it necessary. Such insensitive treatment did not have the desired effect on the quiet lad from the North of England.

> If I had a fancied ride Toby would start on at me first thing in the morning on the gallops and never leave me alone all day. Some people ride better when they are wound up. I don't. I always felt more confident in a race when I knew he wasn't watching me. At Toby's you tended to get a bollocking, win or lose. That demoralized me. He didn't intend to depress me but that's what happened.

Already the problem of excess weight was proving a nuisance for Bob. Tall, at five feet nine, thick set and heavy boned, he had always enjoyed his food and found the idea of not eating singularly unappealing. Clive Bailey remembers how Bob's attempts at wasting and sweating to make the correct racing weights were erratic, unhealthy and sometimes dangerous: "When he was trying to do light he'd come in for breakfast, wolf down two egg sandwiches and follow that with a large tin of fruit. He'd miss out the main meal in the day then in the evening eat three Mars bars and several ice-creams. The joke was that he thought he was a dedicated jockey, trying seriously to lose weight."

On other occasions Bob would go out at night for a meal and a bottle of wine, then spend hours in a sauna the next day trying to boil away unwanted pounds. Soon he was introduced to diuretics, or piss pills as they are known by jockeys for obvious reasons. Diuretics are commonly prescribed for women who suffer from water retention before menstruation, and one pill can cause the loss of three or four pounds of excess fluid in a few hours. Jockeys who take diuretics have to stop every half an hour or so on the way to the races to satisfy the call of nature. At least one rider had to jump off his horse down at the start of a race and pop behind a hedge while he relieved himself. Diuretics are an effective way of losing a few pounds rapidly but the side effects can be devastating. The pills cause sickness, weakness and can seriously damage the functions of the body. Bob used them as a last resort in his early days as a jockey and recalls:

As a short term measure they seemed ideal but I soon found that I was putting back on twice as much in the evening as I had lost in the morning. Sometimes I felt so weak when I'd taken them that I was little more than a passenger on the horses I rode.

Exercising racehorses at home is not the safest of occupations. Young thoroughbreds, freshly broken, can be wild, unsafe conveyances. Bob was chosen as the regular rider of one young chestnut which was so mad that it never ran on a racecourse. Each day he would take the horse out on its own on the country lanes for an hour or two. One morning, as they returned from exercise, Bob, as usual, took his feet out of the stirrup irons as he prepared to jump down and lead the horse the rest of the way home. The horse bolted down the narrow village street, squeezed between a tractor and bus on the sharp bend, swept past the local pub at a pace which seemed to his hapless rider to be well in excess of thirty miles an hour and galloped straight into a river. Bob, who had been clinging on desperately and was, he says, far too frightened to jump off, was catapulted into a bed of mud. Horse and rider were hosed down together much to the amusement of the other lads.

The infamous Swiss Knight was another horse in the yard with alarming habits. Twice in a fortnight he ran away with Bob on the gallops, and a course of solitary exercise was prescribed by Toby Balding to calm the horse down. Bob would disappear on the horse each summer morning for up to two hours. Several people in the stable wondered why Swiss Knight returned without any sweat marks at all, even on the warmest July days. Bob explains:

We used to walk and trot to the pub in the next village of Kimpton. I would tie up Swiss Knight behind the pub, order a half pint of shandy and sit out in the garden reading the *Sporting Life*. That might sound a bit deceitful but Swiss Knight had already shown he was a kinky devil without any brakes and I had no intention of letting him out of control on the roads.

Brain Blister was yet another equine lunatic trained by Toby Balding. One summer morning he ran away with Bob and deposited him in the biggest blackthorn hedge in Hampshire. Bob, who had been wearing a short sleeved shirt, was stuck on the peak of the hedge for several minutes before help arrived and spent the next few weeks on the agonizing task of removing all the particularly painful black-thorns from his body.

By mid-April 1968 Bob had ridden eight winners and was fourth in the list of successful amateurs behind the runaway leader Richard Tate. In those days the Jockey Club issued A and B amateur permits. Once a jockey had ridden ten winners he had to appear before the licensing stewards to prove that he was a genuine amateur and so was qualified to receive a B permit. In Bob's case the stewards decided to interview him after his sixtieth ride. The meeting in London on 20th April lasted fifteen minutes and proved both embarrassing and infuriating for him. The stewards asked Bob to explain how he could afford to continue riding as an amateur. He explained his position as Toby Balding's farm manager.

"But what exactly do you do?" queried one of the stewards.

"I look after the gallops," said Bob, already rattled by the line of questioning.

"But what do you do on the gallops?" the steward persisted.

"Mow and tread in divots."

"What else do you do on the farm?" continued another steward.

"I collect the eggs," answered the young jockey in desperation.

"How many chickens does Mr Balding keep?"

"Five, I think," replied Bob lamely.

Clearly the stewards, guardians of the Corinthians, did not believe the story of Bob's amateur status. They ruled that he had been working for Toby Balding for payment and that this infringed his amateur status and so withdrew his licence to ride. Bob left the interview in despair, without a riding licence of any kind; for over two weeks he was unable to continue his emerging career as a jockey. Toby Balding, astonished at the outcome, made a special trip to Newmarket to appeal to the stewards on his jockey's behalf. Finally, on 6th May, they relented and issued Bob with a professional licence although he insists,

At the time that was the last thing I wanted because I didn't think I was good enough to be offered paid rides. But everything worked out all right in the end. I never did like chickens.

On 13th May 1968, after an absence of almost a month, Bob was given his first chance as a professional jockey on Toby Balding's Sailor's Collar at Wye. They won in style.

Wye, a tight, tiny, sharp racecourse in the depths of Kent, clearly suited Bob, although he was virtually alone in his praise of its doubtful pleasures. On a wet day it was little safer than an ice rink. Multiple pile-ups were part of the regular entertainment there and the sheep wire which was spread along under the running rail provided an additional hazard. Aly Branford, knocked out in an ugly fall, was jerked back to consciousness by the horrifying throbbing of a live electric sheep wire wrapped around his arm. Brough Scott, now a television commentator and racing journalist, recalls with wry humour the day he lay trapped in the same wire as the field pounded round the bend towards him. "Riding at Wye," Brough says, "was quite the most dangerous thing anyone could imagine. Down at the start we used to rev up our horses just like motorbikes because if you didn't get off in front you were far more likely to be brought down by the inevitable pile-ups on the bends."

One particularly horrid fall at Wye left Brough unable to move, let alone walk. Bob Champion and Gardie Grissell carried him to the racecourse station and on to the London-bound train. Brough lay immobile on the floor in a carriage that looked as if it had just returned from the battle-front in war time. Bob remembers the occasion well.

It had been an unusually bad day there. Apart from Brough there were several walking wounded with broken collar bones and other minor injuries. When we reached London, Gardie and I loaded Brough into a taxi, gave the driver a fiver and told him to take him to Alun Thomas's clinic in Park Street.

Alun Thomas, a marvellously sympathetic and effective specialist, examined Brough and diagnosed a broken vertebra in his neck. He spent the next month in hospital.

Wye closed down soon after those appalling ordeals. Bob Champion, who was leading jockey at the course for several seasons, viewed the decision with immense regret:

I loved the place. If you went round Wye and gave up the outside to nobody you would always gain ground because your horse would always be balanced. All right, it was a bit dangerous when it rained and there would be a lot of fallers on the bends but I wish we still raced there.

Chapter 3

BEFORE HIS ILLNESS Bob had made several attempts in the Grand National without success, but at least he could fairly claim that he had ridden a winner of the race. The horse was Highland Wedding, a marvellous old character who was only two weeks from his twelfth birthday when Bob rode him in public for the first time on 14th December 1968 in an important race at Chepstow. The horse had shown little form in the previous twelve months and at Chepstow his regular jockey, Owen McNally, was out of action with an injury. Highland Wedding and his new jockey finished a close third in a competitive race. This was clearly an improvement on previous form, but Bob's hopes of keeping the mount were dashed when the brilliant Irish horseman Eddie Harty replaced him at Ascot where Highland Wedding won. Neither Owen McNally nor Eddie Harty was available on 1st February 1969, when Highland Wedding was sent north for Newcastle's Eider Chase, one of the most important staying races in the calendar. So Bob Champion was re-united with Highland Wedding, who had won the race in 1966 and 1967—and would probably have done so again in 1968 if bad weather had not caused the meeting to be abandoned.

It was Bob's first ride at Newcastle but he gave himself every opportunity of learning the course. In the morning he walked round with fellow jockey Clive Bailey and then completed a second lap with Toby Balding. The trainer had been appalled by photographs of Bob in all the morning papers. The pictures showed Bob clearing the last fence brilliantly at Kempton on the previous day. Unfortunately Time is Money, the horse he had been riding, was standing still on the take-off side. The horse's blinkered head was captured peering through the top of the birch to see what had happened to his jockey. That morning Bob had been asleep in his hotel room when

Toby Balding burst in clutching the morning papers, spread them over the bed and insisted he did not want the same thing happening to Highland Wedding.

The going at Newcastle was soft, almost heavy, testing conditions for the toughest of stayers, but even so Highland Wedding started a warm favourite to complete a famous hat-trick. Bob rode a patient, waiting race, moved easily into the lead with a mile left and came to the last fence with the race already won. But that final obstacle so nearly caused their downfall. No doubt tiring in the sticky ground Highland Wedding misjudged the fence, hit it hard and for one ghastly moment threatened to dislodge his jockey. But Bob sat admirably tight and together they came back to a fine reception. Bob recalls the race:

He jumped brilliantly throughout and the only reason he made that mistake at the last fence was because I had Toby's warning on my mind. I knew I had to get over it in one piece. I'd been giving him a kick into his fences all the way but this time I froze, left him alone and was too careful altogether. He got too close, hit the top, arched his back and landed steep but I never thought I'd come off him.

Toby Balding told a clutch of waiting reporters. "Bob is going to be a very good jockey indeed. He's such a natural horseman."

Now Highland Wedding was right on course for a third and final attempt at the Grand National. But would his eager young jockey be given the chance of a lifetime at Liverpool? Eventually Toby Balding preferred the experience of Eddie Harty, who had once ridden for Ireland in the Olympics, and Bob watched the race a little forlornly on television at Fyfield as Highland Wedding and Eddie Harty drew clear of Steel Bridge on the run-in at the end of the 1969 Grand National. Understandably he regarded the win with mixed emotions.

Obviously I was delighted for the horse and the yard, but there was also a feeling of what might have been. If I'm honest I must admit that I don't think I was experienced enough at the time to have done him justice at Liverpool. I'd never ridden there and was still very much a learner, but I would still have liked the chance on him.

Bob's third ride on Highland Wedding, however, proved a dismal anti-climax. The horse was due to retire but seemed so well that Toby Balding decided to give him one final run in the Midlands Grand National at Uttoxeter a month later. Highland Wedding started favourite but after only two fences it was clear to his jockey that his exertions at Liverpool had left their mark:

Any horse who finishes in the Grand National has a hard race, even if they don't show any outward signs of it. The winner usually has the hardest race of all. I was on a hiding to nothing at Uttoxeter. The old horse was clearly not himself so I pulled him up as soon as I could without being lynched.

Bob ended the season with fifteen winners, a perfectly reasonable score in his first full season as a professional in such a competitive stable. But the next three years proved how tough a jump jockey's life can be. After twenty-five wins he was no longer entitled to claim a weight allowance to compensate for his inexperience and had to compete on level terms with the best in the country. He continued working as a stable lad for Toby Balding, up at dawn, summer and winter, mucking out several horses, exercising at least three each day, then returning to the stables in the afternoon to groom three or four until six in the evening. Rides were few and far between. His earnings dropped, and two falls at Christmas put him out of action for five weeks. By the end of the next season, in June 1970, his winning tally had reached only ten. Doubts about his future began to occupy his mind. Should he perhaps, after all, have continued his farming career with his uncle?

At least a series of girlfriends helped lift the gloom and a holiday in the sun strengthened his resolve to give himself one more season. He returned to Toby Balding's in July fit, bronzed and ready for the new campaign, and then, two days before the opening meeting at Newton Abbot, he broke his left ankle again in an identical fall to the one he suffered when he first joined the stable. This time the culprit was a useless novice chaser named Pieces. The horse had just returned into training after a summer at grass. As Bob was legged into the saddle the horse went berserk, threw him and kicked him, shattering his left ankle. He lay in agony five yards away from the spot where Dozo had broken the same ankle three years earlier. This time he was taken to Winchester Hospital where the break was set in plaster.

Grumbling at his luck, miserable at missing the first months of the season, Bob moped around Toby Balding's office, waiting impatiently for the break to mend. He spent some time on the farm as he was still able to drive a tractor. He even persuaded the stable blacksmith to make an unusually large stirrup iron to accommodate his left leg encased in plaster, and rode out in discomfort for two days until his doctor gave him a serious lecture on the folly of his actions. He admits he was not pleasant company during that time.

I put on weight, got on everyone's nerves and made a right nuisance of myself. There were times when I felt like packing the whole thing in but the truth is I've never found anything in life to rival the feeling of racing at speed over fences. I've never been interested in anything other than racing and each day while I was injured seemed to drag on for forty-eight hours. I was impossible to live with.

He was passed fit to ride again on the last day of October but he had to wait another ten barren weeks before his first win on You're Lucky at Nottingham on 12th January 1971. It was his first victory for eleven months. A more important success came on the little mare Country Wedding at Taunton early in March which prompted Toby Balding to run her in the Grand National.

Every jump jockey's ambition is to ride in the Grand National. Although small, Country Wedding was a sensible jumper, a dour stayer and had the benefit of the same sire as Highland Wedding. Bob spent the week before the race living in the local sauna bath. He ate little and eventually reduced his weight to the required ten stone.

I was quite pleased with myself. I've not managed ten stone many times in my life. I wasted bloody hard in the usual way: sweating and physics—that's to say laxatives that have you sitting on the lavatory for hours. We stayed in Chester and I rode out in the morning. Breakfast? You *must* be joking. Half a cup of coffee, that's all.

Later that morning he walked round the course that he had seen before only on television.

The fences were not quite as big as I'd expected. People had been jumping them for over a hundred years so I couldn't see why it should be different for me. The first ditch frightened me more than any of the others. It was enormous, a high, solid fence with a huge ditch in front of it. I suppose I'd have jumped things as big out hunting.

He paused before adding thoughtfully, "But not at racing pace."

The atmosphere at the Grand National meeting as the time for the big race approaches is unique. The tension for many participants and their friends and families is at times unbearable. Preliminaries before the race seem to last for ever, and in the jockeys' room a curious change in personality affects many of the riders. Men who are usually the life and soul of any party sit silently staring fixedly at the floor, while others like Bob Champion, who is normally quiet and reserved, talk non-stop. Everyone is nervous before the race; it's more an awareness of the unrivalled pressure than fear at what might happen. Valets, overworked by the presence of so many jockeys in the same race, rush round fixing mufflers, checking saddles, murmuring words of comfort and support.

Fully twenty-five minutes before the race the jockeys filed out nervously to the paddock, some smiling bravely, others grim faced. Bob felt tense in those last, tingling minutes in the paddock and during the subsequent parade in front of the stands, even though Country Wedding was largely ignored in the betting at 50-1.

It was a strange feeling because I was riding in the race without a chance at all. Country Wedding didn't even jump little fences that well. She had no scope and no chance whatsoever of winning or getting round. None. Toby's orders were just to go out and enjoy myself. I thought I'd be a clever jockey for once in my life. I knew my mare wouldn't have the speed to go along with the leaders, so I decided to track Terry Biddlecombe on the previous year's winner Gay Trip. He, at least, was certain to jump round safely.

Down at the start while last minute adjustments were made to girths and stirrups Bob tailed Terry Biddlecombe doggedly. Wherever Gay Trip moved Country Wedding was but a few paces behind. After an interminable delay the starter finally shouted, "Go on then," the tapes rose and thirty-eight of the world's toughest steeplechasers thundered away, fanning out in a cavalry charge as they sought a clear approach to the first fence. Gay Trip was just behind and to the outside of the leaders with Country Wedding on his heels. The run to the first fence in the Grand National is unusually long, and by the time they reach it the leading horses are often going much faster than their jockeys would wish.

Country Wedding, in the second wave, met the fence perfectly, soared over it, landed on Gay Trip who had already fallen, and somersaulted, ejecting her jockey like a spent cartridge. Bob lay rolled up tightly, his hands instinctively protecting his head from careless hooves until the field had swept by, and then found he was one of five jockeys who had come down at the first fence.

They trudged disconsolately the few hundred yards back to the stands to watch the field jump the water on the first circuit and then the finish a few minutes later. Bob was inconsolable. "I can't believe it," he kept muttering as, unscathed, he sat miserably in the weighing-room in his muddy silks. At last he mustered some sort of joke. "At least I was going well when I fell," he offered weakly as his valet, Robin Lord, pulled off his boots, and ten years later he still remembers the acute disappointment.

Gay Trip fell and brought me down. My mare went straight over the top of Terry's horse and turned arse over head. When she came down I wanted the race to be stopped, wound back and re-run so that we could join in again. The thought of waiting another whole year for a second chance was too agonizing to consider.

The final weeks of the season proved unbearably dull after Liverpool. Bob ended the season with a mere eight winners, his lowest total yet. In four years' honest endeavour he had managed just forty-three winning rides and was no nearer to achieving his declared ambition to finish among the top ten jockeys.

Even so, his win in the Eider Chase the previous year and his ride in the Grand National, however brief, had brought him to the attention of his old school, the Laurence Jackson School at Guisborough. In the summer he was surprised and a little alarmed to be invited back there to open the summer fete. He drove to Yorkshire while on holliday, persuaded Derek Thompson's mother to write a small speech for him and arrived at the school in his unaccustomed role of VIP. Making the speech proved a terrifying ordeal but soon he had shaken off the polite attentions of his former masters and disappeared among the sidestalls. There, to his intense delight, he found a stall that offered two shillings to anyone accurate enough to burst three balloons at three attempts with a bow and arrow. He recalls with much relish:

As you know I was useless at school, but one thing I could use was a bow and arrow. This stall was just like taking money from the bank every few minutes. The balloons were so close that I couldn't miss. In the end it became embarrassing so I collected my ill-gotten gains and let someone else have a go. No, I wasn't asked back again.

That summer was also memorable for a week's fasting before a visit to Ostend where he won the Prix Fabien Hurdle on Toby Balding's Wide World. He shed almost a stone in seven days using harsh, unwise methods and spent the next day regretting his actions.

A holiday in Ibiza with Derek Thompson also provided some light relief. They worked as a highly skilled duo. Bob, a dedicated sunbather, would patrol the beaches during the day, arranging dates for both of them each night. In the evenings, while Bob slept, Derek emerged to canvass the likeliest bars and clubs for possible talent. Often they would be double-booked and eventually it became less demanding to stay with the same girls. They settled for two policewomen from Bolton, who they first saw taking part in a Miss Hawaii competition. The boys returned home a week early, exhausted by their activities.

"Bob has this curious attraction for women," says Derek. "He's unlike anyone else I've met. He's quiet, doesn't say very much and is definitely shy but somehow they flock round him. Perhaps it's the twinkle in his eye. When he does talk to them he tends to be rude and the funny thing is that they keep coming back for more. Even so he's never been a playboy. Race riding always comes first, but as soon as the day's racing is over he calls in on a succession of women. I've never seen such a fast operator."

Bob's fascination clearly did not work the night he and Derek took out two girls in London. After dinner at the Playboy Club they moved on to a nightclub in the King's Road. Finally it was time to go home and Bob sat in the back seat of Derek's car with his arms cosily round the girl he had met only that night. When Derek stopped to drop her off at her home Bob, too, climbed out clutching his suitcase, followed her to the front door and was furious when she shut it in his face. Eventually she did press the buzzer to open the door and Bob pounded eagerly up the stairs to her flat. But that door was locked, too, and despite his pleas and eventual threats she, wise girl, refused to let him in. So he charged back down the stairs and into the street in the faint hope that Derek might still be waiting there. It was too late. The time was three a.m. and so Bob wandered angrily along the streets of Bayswater with his suitcase until he found a seedy hotel that was open. He was still fuming the next morning.

Bob's luck in the 1971–72 season was not much better. He managed just ten winners and another ride in the Grand National on Country Wedding. Again they started at 50-1. Bob stayed in a hotel at Southport, enjoyed a night out with several other jockeys and spent the morning of the race in the sauna on the seafront sipping champagne as he shed a few ounces of excess weight. The session in the sauna on Grand National morning has become something of a ritual for the jockeys. It's a way of relieving the tension, losing weight and avoiding the endless stream of well-wishers, journalists, strangers and others who tend to pester them in the hours before the race. Bob ended up carrying four pounds overweight at 10 stone

4 pounds. but it didn't make any difference. Country Wedding negotiated the first fence safely this time and was going well enough, though towards the rear, when she fell at the eleventh.

That year, for the briefest of spells, Bob found to his surprise and trepidation that he was retained jockey for the most formidable of women trainers of the day. This particular woman undoubtedly had a talent for training racehorses but she also had the ability to swear like a trooper, shout in the gravelly tones of a sergeant-major and run down jockeys publicly in scathing tones. Bob won races for her at Worcester and Plumpton, but their brief partnership came to an abrupt conclusion the day he made the serious tactical error of agreeing to school her horse over her own fences at home. As soon as the horse he was riding did something wrong, the trainer began bawling at Bob in the foulest possible language. His reaction to such a verbal onslaught should be in the text books for all budding jockeys. He jumped off the horse, let go of the reins and told her icily, "If you don't like it ride the horse yourself", strode to his car and drove off leaving her, for once, open mouthed and speechless.

Despite that entertaining interlude his career as a jockey seemed to be faltering. Most of the horses he was riding had no possible chance of winning. Some were bad jumpers, many were simply too slow. Good rides were not being offered to him. Bob sums up:

For five years I rode for Toby Balding, looked after my horses in the yard and did all sorts of odd jobs around the stables. I rode ten winners in my first season and ten in my fifth season and that could hardly be called progress. I thought I was riding better but I was still back at square one. There were too many jockeys in the stable and so we were all struggling for rides. I was making a safe, if small, living by working in the yard as well but I was barely able to save anything by the time I paid for all my expenses such as my car, telephone, valet fees and medical bills.

It didn't seem at all likely that I would ever become first jockey at Fyfield. Toby hardly helped my confidence by bollocking me all the time, even though he was great fun to be with after racing. He was always generous and looked after us at clubs and restaurants on the way home, but I felt part of the furniture and couldn't see a future for myself there.

So after five years, Bob left Toby Balding and decided to make the best of his opportunities as a freelance. After a holiday in Cyprus he moved in with his sister Mary, by then married to Richard Hussey, a farmer who lived on the outskirts of Wootton Bassett near Swindon. Bob helped on the farm and wondered how he would find rides in the early months of the new season.

Mary and Bob's girlfriend Sarah ploughed their way through a list of local racing stables looking for a trainer who might need a jockey. One of their choices was Monty Stevens, an interesting character who had recently bought Lucknam Park near Chippenham in Wiltshire and was in the process of converting it into a racing stable. Bob spoke to Monty's son Jeffrey at the races, arranged to ride out there the following morning and within three days was offered a retainer.

Monty Stevens, who died in 1977, was a man of the country. He made a fortune as a farmer and cattle breeder and fashioned the seven hundred acre Lucknam Park estate into a racing paradise. He began by founding a stud there and then in the summer of 1972, without any previous experience at all, started training his own horses with instant success. At the time Bob joined Monty in July 1972, the number of horses he trained—twenty-three—matched, by coincidence, the total of bedrooms in his massive house.

Monty Stevens relied heavily on instinct, and as he watched Bob ride out the first morning he realized he was a natural horseman. Monty had no practical experience of racing and preferred to rely on a fund of knowledge, understanding and feeling for animals. It did not occur to him that he might not succeed as a trainer and he didn't bother to go racing to see his horses run. Instead he tended to sit in the comfort of his enormous living-room listening to the betting shop commentary piped through to his home. Bob's third ride for Monty Stevens was on Winden at the start of the new jump season at Devon and Exeter on 3rd August. They won by twelve lengths. More winners for the stable followed, other trainers began to use Bob and for the first time in his life he was in demand. The decision to leave Toby Balding, delayed for so long, had clearly been correct and overdue.

Bob's victory on the headstrong mare Squiffy in a modest steeple-chase at Wye early in October made headlines in all the racing papers. The official form book, in its time-honoured brief style, merely reported, "Squiffy, R. Champion, led third fence, soon clear, easily." Behind this terse statement lay a remarkable feat of horsemanship. Squiffy, insists Bob, was lacking in two essential qualities demanded by any sensible jockey: brakes and steering.

> She was crazy, daft and no-one could hold her. After jumping two fences she was always miles in front of the others. Your only chance was to sit tight and wait until she settled.

A mile or so from home, when Squiffy still held a clear lead, the buckle on one of Bob's stirrup leathers broke and the weight of his feet on it caused the iron to plunge to the ground. Bob lurched for one perilous second on to Squiffy's neck, then kicked out his other foot from the remaining iron to preserve his balance. Dr David Chesney, the dashing young amateur in distant pursuit on Less Curious, looked ahead and thought, "My God, Bob's riding longer than ever today!"

Bob's position, however, was far from amusing with a complete circuit of the tight Wye course to negotiate. Jockeys in such situations have three options: to try to pull up, to risk jumping off, or to bash on in the remote hope of crossing the remaining fences without falling off. Wye was hardly the ideal place to attempt a rodeo show but, as Bob explains, he had no alternative.

> She was going far too fast to pull up and I don't know of a jockey brave enough to jump off so I had no choice but to continue riding without irons. Squiffy could be very ignorant at some of her fences but thank goodness this time she was fine until she tried to walk through the second last. I was sitting so far back I managed to stay on, she jumped the last well and we won easily by fifteen lengths. My share of the prize money was £27 and that didn't really make up for the pain and inconvenience of the next few days. I was incredibly sore and could hardly walk.

Bob's ride in the Grand National that season was a total outsider, Hurricane Rock, once a useful chaser in the north of England but a horse who had lost all his form since joining his new trainer, Desmond Dartnall. Hurricane Rock started at 100-1 but anyone spirited enough to back him in the weeks before the race would have had no trouble in finding bookmakers to oblige him at 500-1. Imagine Bob Champion's surprise, then, when he moved into third place with three fences to go. Hurricane Rock was still third over the final fence but he tired badly and finished sixth to the immortal Red Rum, who was winning the first of his three Grand Nationals. Bob recalls that day:

> When Brian Fletcher made his move on Red Rum I tried to go with him but Hurricane Rock was just not good enough. We kept third place for a while over the last three fences but Hurricane Rock was legless on the run-in and almost stopped to a walk. Even so to finish sixth was the biggest thrill I ever had, more so because no one gave the horse any chance at all.

A month later the death of Doug Barrott came as a brutal reminder of the darker side of jump racing. Doug, a bright, cheerful character, was stable jockey to Josh Gifford and died when French Colonist fell in the Whitbread Gold Cup at Newcastle. Doug, like all his friends in the weighing-room, readily accepted the hazards of riding over fences, a spectacle that gives so much entertainment to millions of followers. Racing was in his blood, the excitement and comradeship of sharing a common danger a powerful and addictive drug. Doug Barrott was the second rider to be killed in six months and the seventh in seven years—unpalatable figures that reveal starkly why jump racing will always be such a dangerous sport.

Chapter 4

BY THE SUMMER of 1973 Bob Champion was established as a tough, competent professional, still considered by many racegoers as more of a horseman than a jockey. Honest, reliable, punctual and hard working, very much the perfectionist, he was extremely confident on a horse and surprisingly reserved, almost self-effacing, on his own two feet. His natural shyness did not, however, prevent him pursuing with enthusiasm, skill and not a little success a legion of warm-eyed females. A curious pastime, you may consider, for a man whose favourite saying was and is, "Women ain't people."

His relationships with his girlfriends tended to be tempestuous, passionate and erratic. When roused the quiet lad from Yorkshire could, at times, reveal a remarkably stubborn—some might say mean and unkind—streak. One delightful girl who matched him admirably and shared his life for a few years was Sarah. She quickly decided that attack was the best form of defence when Bob was in an obstinate, impossible mood. Once while they stood arguing on the stands at Newton Abbot races, she thrust an ice-cream up his nose. "The cone and all," one amused observer reported later.

Jim Old, a close friend of Bob and Sarah's from the days at Fyfield, had started training in a farmyard next to a duckpond in the remote Dorset village of Ashmore. Bob and Sarah were regular visitors at weekends and holidays and would help straighten the place out. On one occasion an argument developed as they took their things out of the car boot. Bob picked Sarah up, dumped her in the boot of the car and despite her screams of protest, locked it and marched into the house.

Jim wanted to let Sarah out but Bob stopped him. "Don't do it," he cried. "She'll go mad and try to kill me!"

After ten minutes or so Bob finally relented, released the catch on the boot and ran as a fiery Sarah, understandably wild with a mixture of fear and fury, leaped out of the car, seized the nearest pitchfork and chased him round the stable yard.

"She was like an angry wasp and I don't blame her," Jim says. "She was set on skewering Bob to the nearest convenient wall." Bob, who had retreated with commendable speed, spotted a bucket of water, hastily picked it up and hurled the contents over his attacker. The water, apparently, had the desired effect though it's difficult to believe Jim's claim that the rest of the weekend passed peacefully at the duckpond.

Jim Old's right hand man and most constant supporter at the time was Sally Thomas, a good natured girl who distrusted men instinctively and thwarted all Jim's considerable charm and persuasive attempts at seduction. Bob, whose own amorous adventures had met only the occasional refusal, could not understand Sally's determined resistance and decided to help his friend achieve his objective. On his next visit to Ashmore he found Jim and Sally painting the inside of a stable. Acting with the spirit of the soft-hearted romantic he certainly is not, he locked and bolted the door and refused to release the couple until they had agreed to marry. A month later Sally became Jim's wife and Bob gained his reward for such astute matchmaking by riding the first of Jim's winners as a trainer, Winged Dagger, at the Devon and Exeter meeting on 8th August 1973.

At home Bob was fanatical about tidiness. He would insist that his girlfriends kept his rooms immaculate and spotless at all times. "You don't keep a dog to bark yourself," he would say. A neat and orderly person he expected everyone else to be equally tidy. One newspaper thrown carelessly on the floor was enough to annoy him. Sometimes, at dinner parties, he would polish the table between courses and usually he ensured that all the washing-up was completed before coffee was served.

Bob had ended the 1972–73 season, his first as a freelance, with twenty-nine wins from 227 rides. Clearly the move had been a success. He started the new season with such a flourish that he led the jockeys' table for the first few weeks. Josh Gifford, without a stable jockey following the death of Doug Barrott, noted Bob's run of success. Josh began the season hoping one of the several young apprentices in his yard would emerge to fill the role of stable jockey, but results in the early months of the season were not encouraging. Some of his owners made it clear they would prefer an experienced jockey on their horses and after a brief search Josh's choice narrowed to Richard Evans and Bob Champion. Both were given chances on the stable's horses.

Bob's first ride for Josh Gifford on Clare Dawn could scarcely have been more disastrous. Clare Dawn, a 16-1 outsider in a three-horse novice chase at Kempton, had fallen in two of her three previous races. This time she came to the last fence in second place, then made a telling mistake which sent her eager jockey tumbling to the ground under her feet.

> I remember lying there thinking I had blown whatever chance I had of landing the job when Josh came running down the track. At least he had the decency to ask me if I was all right before helping me back into the saddle.

The judge waited patiently in his box until Clare Dawn and her bruised jockey eventually stumbled across the line to qualify for third place money. Four days later Bob won on Captain Hardy for Josh Gifford at Windsor. Other rides and winners followed, and Josh soon offered him a retainer for the following season.

> It honestly was an offer I couldn't refuse. I'd been messing around mostly on bad horses for the previous six or seven years and now I had the chance to ride for one of the most promising young trainers in the country.

Josh Gifford explains the reasons he chose Bob Champion: "The best jockey is the one who has the fewest falls and it was clear Bob was a superb horseman. Jumping is the name of the game. If horses jump they are going to win races. A race is won from the time the starting gate goes up, out in the country, by a sympathetic rider who gets them round in the most economic way. Also Bob was not a man who resorted to the whip very often. I'm against whip jockeys. A jockey who rides with a sensible length of stirrup doesn't have to use the stick too much. Remember if a horse doesn't go for one or two cracks he's not going to go for twelve."

No man is better qualified to air his views on the subject. Josh Gifford, a dynamic jockey, started riding on the flat at the age of eleven, was one of the most successful apprentices of his era, switched to jump racing when he became too heavy and was champion jockey four times. He retired in April 1970 after his final ride in the Grand National and began training at Findon just a few miles from Worthing in Sussex.

The next five seasons proved fruitful years for the new partnership. Bob continued to live in Wiltshire, at first sharing a house in Hungerford with fellow jockey John Haine and later renting two more with a girlfriend before buying his own home in a quiet village near Hungerford in March 1977. He would drive to Findon a dozen times a season at Josh's request to school a particular horse over hurdles or fences and would sometimes stay overnight for one of the local meetings at Plumpton or Fontwell. Says Josh, "The only other times we saw him here were when he wanted a bed and obviously was in need of a rest from all his girlfriends."

Weight was a constant problem and hunger an unwelcome companion. For a time Bob joined John Haine and that notable weight watcher Terry Biddlecombe in regular morning sessions at the Turkish Baths in Gloucester. Terry, tall and flamboyant, epitomized the unquenchable spirit of jump jockeys. His friendly nature and legendary zest for all that is best in life made his never-ending struggle with the scales all the more difficult to endure. The three friends would sit in the Turkish Baths, steaming gently, at a time when most citizens of Gloucester were still in bed. Then they would drive to the races and Biddlecombe, still anxious to shed even more weight, would sometimes wear a rubber sweat suit under several sets of clothes with the car heater on.

Bob became so desperate to reduce his weight that he visited a London doctor notorious for providing drastic slimming aids. The doctor used a harsh method to suit the needs of his racing patients—injections followed by a series of amphetamine pills. The injection, a powerful diuretic, caused dehydration, the loss of existing body liquid and a brief but rapid drop in weight. The pills contained an effective stimulant which speeded up the system and also dulled the usual pangs of hunger. Most of the doctor's patients seemed to be wafer-thin models trying desperately to retain their sylph-like figures. Jockeys were merely occasional extras in his consulting room. After a brief examination Bob was given a single injection in his backside and two boxes of pills, one of each to be taken every day. Bob, who is prone on occasions to exaggerate, claims,

> That injection nearly killed me. I talked to the doctor for a few minutes after it, limped out of the surgery and struggled towards my car as my legs started to seize up. I've never known so much pain. I passed out in the street. Luckily a policeman helped me to my car where I sat for two hours pouring sweat. I felt like death.

Eventually he felt able to drive himself home. He took the pills for about a week then stopped because they made him feel so ill.

> I believe they are usually given to heart patients and are designed to make you feel on top of the world. Well, they had the opposite effect on me. They were sending me mental. I behaved very strangely in that week. I couldn't sleep, couldn't see properly, was driving dangerously and my reflexes were a lot slower. I felt just as bad riding in a race.

After that alarming experience Bob reverted to the two more traditional methods jockeys use to lose weight in a hurry—piss pills and saunas. One pill taken in the morning would ensure he lost three or four pounds in the next few hours.

> At first I had to stop frequently for a pee on the way to the races but then I made sure I took the pills earlier in the morning. But as usual I put on twice as much weight afterwards. Sometimes they would make me feel weak though you only realized it at the end of a race. Sometimes, too, I used to get attacks of cramp in my hands.
>
> I also used various laxative pills which were an even more dire way of shedding unwanted pounds. The pills are to relieve

constipation. We take them when we are not constipated. The effect of that is a sort of self-induced constant Spanish tummy. Some jockeys try Exlax, a laxative produced in the form of chocolate. I couldn't face the stuff. I found it quite horrible. I intended to try it two or three times but just a taste of it was enough to make me feel sick.

On 25th October 1975, Bob Champion won on all four of his rides in successive races at Huntingdon. The quartet—Man on the Moon, Blue Bidder, Captain George and Clare Dawn—were all trained by Josh Gifford. It was a tremendous feat by both trainer and jockey but such are the fluctuations of fortune in jump racing that Bob fell heavily on his next mount, I Picture You, at the first hurdle at Plumpton.

By the mid-seventies he was unable to ride at less than ten and a half stone without a few days' warning. One Christmas, readers of a large circulation magazine were to be seen with tears in their eyes after a story appeared outlining the awful deprivation suffered by Bob Champion over the festive season. Female hearts pined in sympathy at the very thought of poor Bob's miserly Christmas Day menu of a lightly boiled egg and a solitary cup of tea while "his wife and two children tucked into a large turkey." This last reference to his family came as a particular shock to his mother and constant girlfriend who, like the rest of us, had noticed his reluctance to give up his bachelor status. The line about the egg was rather more accurate.

Each year there was always the dream of winning the Grand National. Although he put up overweight in 1975 he finished sixth on Manicou Bay, his first National ride for Josh Gifford. The following year he completed the race once more, though well down the field, on Money Market. John Burke, a friend who changed next to him, won that Grand National on Rag Trade and Bob could hardly refuse the constant supply of champagne in the heady moments after the race. Both jockeys were due to ride in the final race of the day, a novice hurdle, and I suspect neither would have passed the breathalyser test as they jogged out to the paddock in a cloud of bubbles. Bob resents any such implication.

I was in command all right. I jumped my horse Charlotson out of the gate in front, we made all the running, held on well on the flat and won comfortably. It was the best ride I've given a horse. Ever.

The 1977 Grand National, for Bob Champion, was a major anti-climax. His mount, the experienced old handicapper Spittin' Image, capsized at the first fence. The next year he fell again, this time at the ninth fence, on Shifting Gold.

In yet another attempt to lessen his weight problems Bob began taking pills that speeded up his metabolism and tended to dull his appetite, but they had unusual side effects.

I lost weight a lot quicker when I first started taking these pills. They speeded up my body and left me terribly bright in the morning but when the effects wore off I would be exhausted. Once you'd taken one you couldn't sleep if you wanted to. The tablets jazzed me up to such an extent that my body was working twice as fast as normal. But at least I didn't want to eat as much as usual.

The mystery of some extra pounds led to a rare carpeting from the Newbury stewards after Bob finished third on Aldaniti in the 1977 Hennessy Cognac Gold Cup. A tough, genuine old-fashioned type of steeplechaser, Aldaniti had been named after the four grandchildren of his breeder Tommy Barron—the first two letters of the names of twins Alastair and David Cook, and of Nicola and Timothy Barron. Foaled in 1970 at Tommy Barron's Harrowgate Stud at Darlington, Aldaniti was unfashionably bred but, curiously, shared the same fifth dam as Grundy, the 1975 Derby winner. That Derby was still more than a year away when Tommy Barron sent Aldaniti to the Ascot Bloodstock Sales in May 1974 where he was bought for 3,200 guineas by Josh Gifford on the advice of his father-in-law George Roger-Smith.

Aldaniti raced in the colours of Josh Gifford's wife, the former showjumper Althea Roger-Smith, when he won easily over hurdles on his racecourse debut at Ascot in January 1975 ridden by Bob. Nick Embiricos, who had horses in training with Josh, had been so impressed with Aldaniti when he had seen him at Findon that he had asked for first refusal if the horse was ever for sale. Soon after that first victory the Giffords duly sold Aldaniti for a reasonable profit to Nick Embiricos, a shipbroker who also ran a small stud with his wife Valda on their farm at Kirdford in Sussex.

Aldaniti did not win again over hurdles and subsequently suffered a serious strain to the tendon on his right foreleg. In racing terms he had broken down on his off fore. A bar firing operation, the traditional method of healing tendon trouble, was carried out before Aldaniti was sent home to the Barkfold Manor Stud at Kirdford for a long rest. He did not race for thirteen months. When he returned into training, apparently cured, he was switched immediately to steeplechasing, a role for which his owners, trainer and jockey all believed he was ideally suited. After an early setback when he unseated Bob at Newbury he won for the first time over fences at Ascot on 1st April 1977, the day before that year's Grand National. Following that easy success he developed rapidly into one of the most promising young chasers in the country and Bob had come back after winning the Leicestershire Silver Fox Chase on him early in November prophesying that the horse would one day win the Grand National.

At Newbury at the end of November Aldaniti was handicapped to carry ten stone in the valuable Hennessy Cognac Gold Cup, one of the most competitive races of the season. That weight, of course, was impossible for Bob but he promised Josh and Nick and Valda Embiricos that he would ride at 10 stone 7 pounds and he duly weighed out at exactly that mark. An almighty blunder by Aldaniti at the second fence almost ended his part in the proceedings but the horse found an extra leg, Bob sat admirably tight and they set off in pursuit of the distant field of runners. Aldaniti recovered so well that he had every chance of winning two fences from home but he could not quicken further and finished a creditable third, beaten by just over three lengths by Bachelors Hall and Fort Devon.

Unfortunately when Bob weighed in immediately after the race the scales remained stubbornly at 10 stone 11 pounds. Horses that finish in the first four are disqualified if their jockeys return appreciably lighter than when they weighed out before a race. The importance to the betting public of overweight, too, means that jockeys are not supposed to come back heavier after a race. What, the Newbury stewards demanded forcibly, was the reason for the extra four pounds? Bob strenuously denied sipping more than a cup of tea between his two appearances on the scales but the stewards did not accept his explanation and warned him to be more careful in future. Jockeys have been known to weigh out in paper cheating boots, carrying a weight cloth without a saddle or stirrup leathers. Did Bob Champion perhaps use this guise to fool the clerk of the scales? He smiles sheepishly and mutters that he cannot remember. His running battle with one clerk of the scales reached such an uncharitable point that once he put two laxatives in the wretched man's tea at the races.

After the extensive publicity that followed Bob's exceptional overweight at Newbury, the stewards of the Jockey Club conducted an exhaustive and quite serious investigation into the precise increase in body weight caused by drinking a cup of tea!

Aldaniti was found to be lame after the Hennessy Cognac Gold Cup. He had chipped two pieces of bone off his pastern just below his fetlock joint on his right hind leg, or off hind, probably when he clouted the second fence so hard. Only his undoubted courage helped him finish the race in such a condition. After a detailed examination Josh Gifford's vet Mike Ashton decided that Aldaniti's sole hope of racing again would be complete rest for at least six months. So the horse returned once more to the Barkfold Manor Stud where he remained restricted to his box from December 1977 until July 1978—an extremely long period of confinement for such an active and enthusiastic racehorse. While he was recovering Aldaniti was in the excellent care of Beryl Millem, head girl at the stud, and her two assistants Lin Wilcox and Margaret Phillips. Time, as usual, proved the best healer of all and the patience of Aldaniti's owners and their staff was amply rewarded when he was led out of his box early in July walking sound again, the breaks on his damaged leg fully mended.

Jockeys are not allowed to bet and are punished severely if they are caught doing so. Many of them use their friends or "punters" to do their betting for them. One retired flat-race jockey was said to have had more "punters" than the Ipswich Town football team had supporters.

Recently a leading jump jockey, riding a hot favourite in a novice hurdle for one of the country's most successful trainers, weighed out at 10 stone 4 pounds and returned a few minutes later, after finishing second, weighing 10 stone 3 pounds.

"You've just lost one pound," the clerk of the scales told him.

"No, you're wrong there," groaned the dejected jockey. "I've just lost £200."

All jockeys have their own medical record books in which racecourse doctors register each injury at the time it happens. Bob's book is full of the usual catalogue of broken ankles, vertebrae, collar bones, ribs, fingers and toes, along with numerous cases of concussion, bruising and lacerations. In December 1977 he suffered one of the worst falls of all from Billet Doux II in a novice chase at Cheltenham. Billet Doux II somersaulted at a downhill fence, fell on his jockey as he landed and brought down another horse who crushed Bob under him. It was a terrifying moment for Bob.

> That was the only time I thought I was dying after a fall. I was knocked out and when I came round I couldn't breathe. I went out again and dreamed I was dead. Then I woke up in the ambulance with an oxygen mask on my face and I knew I would be all right. I felt as though I had been under a steam roller, as if the horse had squeezed the very last ounce of breath out of me. But I was lucky. I only broke a shoulder and some ribs.

Despite increasing weight problems which restricted the number of horses he could ride, Bob ended the 1977–78 season with 56 winners, the best total of his career. Only the champion Jonjo O'Neill and John Francome won more races. Josh Gifford, too, enjoyed his best season with 82 winners. After four years their partnership was an outstanding success.

The Gifford stable held a prolonged celebration at the end of the season to mark the extraordinary feat of the American George Sloan becoming the British amateur jockeys' champion with 23 wins. Sloan owns health spas in Nashville, Tennessee, employs five hundred people, trains his own horses there and runs the Hillsboro' Foxhounds from his fourteen hundred acre estate. A group of fourteen friends, known as the Tennessee Jubilee Sports Syndicate, raised 275,000 dollars towards his costs for the year, purchased a string of useful horses in England, kept most of them with Josh Gifford and got much of their money back by selling the horses at the end of a triumphant campaign. They reduced their costs further by backing George to win the title at lucrative odds.

His victory complete, George invited Bob Champion to America during the summer break. Bob flew to the United States for the first time in May with a friend, Hugo Bevan, clerk of the course, raconteur and unpaid Public Relations Officer for the Playboy Club.

The visitors were welcomed into a very rich American society where, Hugo reports with a trace of envy, the US matrons immediately took Bob to their hearts. "There was something about his quiet, modest manner that made him an immense hit there with the ladies and he became popular with everyone."

Bob took every opportunity that was going to establish himself as a jockey in America. Within a day of arriving he started riding work for local trainers and would go jogging on most mornings to ensure his weight stayed at a sensible level.

"The locals in Tennessee thought he was barmy," Hugo says. "Talk about mad dogs and Englishmen. He would go out running in the burning midday sun. Once while he was out we fiddled the scales he was using. He came back pouring sweat thinking he'd lost a lot of weight and found he'd actually put on a pound. He was livid."

Bob became an expert at operating the citizens'-band radio, known as CB, used by so many American motorists. This system is employed by truck drivers and others for communication and to warn fellow motorists when police patrol cars are in the vicinity.

Says Hugo: "You have to remember there was a speed limit of 55 miles an hour at the time. Bob would be steaming down the highway at a hundred in a car he'd borrowed from a beautiful and wealthy young admirer. He'd have one hand on the wheel and the other working the two-way radio. His call sign was Jockey. He'd be talking to cars coming from the other direction finding out where all the police cars were stationed. The call sign for patrol cars was

Smokey Bear. The only trouble was that most Americans in the deep South couldn't understand his accent as he spoke too quickly."

The duo spent a riotous holiday at first with George Sloan and later with other equally generous hosts, and Bob liked America so much that he accepted an invitation to remain in the country for the summer as a paid work rider, exercising horses each morning on racetracks. He met Jonathan Sheppard, an English trainer doing well there, and stayed with an American jockey Tommy Skiffington who had ridden in England in the early seventies. Bob agreed to work for Burly Cocks, a veteran trainer based in Unionville, Pennsylvania.

Bob soon discovered that jump racing is very much the poor relation to the flat in America. Races are few and far between as punters, quite reasonably, do not like risking their money on horses that might fall. Even so the value of prize money for the limited number of jump races there is lavish by English standards, and when Burly Cocks's regular jockey was not available Bob was delighted to accept a ride in a race at Delaware. The horse finished fourth, but the quiet young Englishman impressed the local trainers so much that he ended the week by riding in four of the five jump races at the Delaware meeting. He won a steeplechase on Wild Sir, trained by Tommy Voss, and was intrigued to share the changing-room with such well known flat-race jockeys as Angel Cordero, Willie Shoemaker and the emerging sensation Steve Cauthen, known universally as "The Kid".

Bob returned to England in August 1978 for the start of the new season but the ground was so firm that Josh Gifford did not intend to run any of his good horses for several weeks. So Bob flew back to America at the request of Tommy Voss, travelled on to Saratoga and in the next month won three more races on Wild Sir. Then it was time to resume his role in England as first jockey to Josh Gifford.

In November Bob gained the biggest victory of his career on Approaching in the Hennessy Cognac Gold Cup. Approaching was handicapped to carry 10 stone 2 pounds—well below his rider's lightest weight. Would another jockey be asked to take over the ride? Wisely Josh Gifford and the horse's owner, Major Derek Wigan, decided Bob's expertise and knowledge of the horse justified putting up several pounds overweight. So began five days of starvation, spent largely at the sauna bath which is included as part of the facilities offered by Hungerford Squash Club. When he is wasting and so missing the pleasure of life, Bob Champion is not the happiest of individuals. As the sweat rolled off so his temper deteriorated. By Saturday morning he was lighter than he had been for years, impossibly hungry and unquestionably grumpy.

His diet that morning was non-existent. Not even a cup of tea before riding out soon after dawn; by nine-thirty he was installed in the racecourse sauna. Boxers in such extreme situations before a big fight have been known to cut their hair, trim their nails and even scrape off a layer of skin from the soles of their feet. Happily that was not deemed necessary for Bob Champion but I imagine Weight Watchers would not have approved of his punishing methods or his wild excesses after his famous victory.

After passing the scales at 10 stone 6 pounds, his lightest for a very long time, he emerged from the racecourse changing-room grey faced and haggard, his pale blue silks hidden under a warm overcoat:

> I've never been so cold in my life. All that wasting causes you to lose your normal resistance to cold. It's the first time I've ever worn a coat in the parade ring. I only hope no-one asks me to do this weight again.

The huge entry for the race had been reduced to eight runners and Bob was able to settle Approaching, four times a course winner, on the inside as Orillo took them along at a swinging gallop. Approaching is not the most spectacular of jumpers. He fell in his first two races over fences and still did not flex his back in the orthodox style for a steeplechaser. But he was so big and nimble that despite the odd fright he seemed to have found a satisfactory method of crossing fences safely. In the Hennessy he was going well throughout and jumped his way to the front six fences from home—sooner than Bob had planned, but he reasoned it seemed sensible to let his horse stride on rather than disappoint him. From that point there was no danger bar a fall. At the last fence he stood way back, gained lengths in the air, landed with the race already won and kept on to beat Master H by five lengths.

Bob's lean and honed features had assumed a constantly miserable guise in the previous forty-eight hours but now he smiled like a man from Death Row who had just earned a reprieve. The starving and wasting were forgotten as he came back on Approaching to a warm reception. Later that night he tucked into a prawn cocktail, steak and salad and then two helpings of his favourite icecream, plus the glasses of champagne that are obligatory on such occasions. On Sunday morning he was suffering from acute stomach ache, though the pain disappeared during the afternoon. He had put on ten pounds.

Bob's victory on Approaching helped him earn numerous bottles of champagne as Bollinger Jockey of the Month for November. An hour after collecting the award Bob was fined a hundred pounds and disqualified from driving for two months for speeding at up to a hundred miles an hour. He was allowed to keep his licence pending an appeal and employed astute delaying tactics so that the appeal was not heard until he had flown to the United States the following May. The appeal failed but by then Bob was in America driving on a licence issued in America.

Approaching was out of action, injured soon after his triumph in the Hennessy, and so Bob rode Aldaniti in the season's most important race, the Cheltenham Gold Cup in March. The race was run in a snowstorm and Bob was delighted to finish third behind the easy winner Alverton. Just over a fortnight later came yet another chance in the Grand National, this time on the New Zealand bred horse Purdo, who led on the inside over the first six fences until falling at Becher's Brook.

It was during the week after the 1979 Grand National that Bob noticed small lumps under each of his nipples. At first he ignored them but when the swelling increased and hardened he drove to London to see Dr Alun Thomas at his clinic just off Park Lane. Alun Thomas, tall, pale and dynamic, had been a mender, supporter and friend of numerous battered jockeys and had patched up Bob a dozen times in the past from a wide variety of injuries. Now he examined the swelling on his breasts and advised him for a while at least to lose weight by sweating in saunas.

The lumps disappeared after little more than a fortnight but Alun Thomas made it clear that Bob should contact him again urgently if they returned.

Chapter 5

THE KICK THAT so dramatically changed Bob Champion's life came without warning at the end of a humdrum novice chase at an evening meeting at Stratford on 11th May 1979. He was riding a promising young chaser, Fury Boy, trained by his friend Nicky Henderson. Bob knew the horse well. He had returned from schooling him over fences two months earlier enthusing, "He's the living best over fences. A natural jumper." That heady opinion was not altered even when he rode Fury Boy at Fontwell on his first outing over fences and they fell at the seventh jump. "He was just a bit too brave, stood off the fence a mile too far and was already coming down when he reached it," Bob explained to Nicky.

Fury Boy duly fulfilled his promise by winning two novice chases and at Stratford was a heavily backed second favourite at 6-4 to complete a hat-trick. Seven horses started in the Brailes Novices' Chase and the risks of riding in such events may well be illustrated by the fact that only two, Fury Boy and Turo, were still standing on the run to the final fence. Fury Boy led there by fully two hundred yards, met it all wrong and crashed to the ground throwing his jockey heavily. Although slightly winded Bob instinctively jumped up and rushed across to the horse who was struggling to his feet. Bob takes up the story:

As I was about to catch him he lashed out with both hind legs and caught me in the balls. It hurt like hell and stopped me for a few seconds but I was too concerned with getting back into the saddle before the other horse came past. I was in agony but I ran alongside Fury Boy, somehow scrambled on to his back, got him going again and still beat Turo by twenty lengths even though I did not find my irons right until the finishing line.

"That was a truly remarkable recovery," Nicky Henderson told reporters huddled in the winner's enclosure. "I think Bob was able to grab the reins because he was quicker on his feet than the horse. Fury Boy is a super jumper but he was so far in front on that last turn that he began to relax and probably the fall was caused by his losing concentration."

Fury Boy proved to be Bob Champion's final winner of the season and the 355th of his career. It was now time for his second summer in America but first he spent a few anxious days worrying about the effects of that unkind kick by Fury Boy.

After that race one of my balls started to swell up for two or three days. It was not so much painful, more a bit numb.

He pauses for a moment, briefly embarrassed, and then adds sheepishly, "Everything was still working all right though. After a few days it seemed perfect again."

Bob flew to America at once, specifically to ride the English trained Casamayor in an international race organized by his friend Hugo Bevan at the Hard Scuffle course on the banks of the Ohio river. Casamayor finished fifth. After an enjoyable weekend at Hard Scuffle Bob moved on to New York for a brief spell as a work rider there, before joining Burly Cocks again in Pennsylvania.

The routine was demanding for anyone unused to waking up so early but work for Bob Champion was finished by ten o'clock on most mornings. Everyone at the stable would be up at six, the horses would be saddled in the big barn by grooms and then Bob and the other work riders would exercise four or five horses each on the sawdust horseshoe-shaped mile-long gallop.

It was a marvellous way of life and I've never felt fitter. The weather was warm and sunny and for the rest of the day we'd go swimming, water skiing, or playing tennis. American hospitality is every bit as good as I'd been led to believe. There were parties every night. I think a "limey" jockey was a bit of a novelty over there.

Race rides this time were scarce but he did win on Obwanknobi at

Monmouth in June. He also found time for a week's holiday at an hotel at Cancun on the Gulf of Mexico where he met an English girl, Nicky, an attractive, dark haired nursing sister who was in America on an exchange course from a hospital in south London that specialized in cancer cases. Bob and Nicky led separate lives during that week but met for a drink sometimes in the evenings.

Bob returned to work for Burly Cocks after a week's break and moved on with the stable's horses for the meeting at Delaware. Jump jockeys are used to knocks, bruises and breaks and do not tend to fuss about the odd bump, but by now Bob was mildly concerned about the swelling that had remained on one of his testicles since he was kicked by Fury Boy back in May.

It was so minor most of the time I didn't think about it but after a while it became more numb. I never dreamed anything was seriously wrong. One of my balls was a little bit firmer than normal but it wasn't uncomfortable in any way. It didn't affect my activities!

A lucky encounter with a vet persuaded him to seek medical advice in England. Why did he ask a vet?

"Well, the vet was there at the time and told me I should catch the next plane back to England and go to see a good doctor."

But why a *vet*?

Bob shuffled his feet. "Well, I was too embarrassed to ask a doctor. The vet was insistent enough for me to take notice and I flew back the next day."

Again. Why question a vet about such a personal matter?

Once more Bob wriggled uncomfortably, before muttering, "Well if you must know she was a female vet and we were in bed at the time."

Bob packed his belongings and on Saturday 21st July flew to Heathrow where he had arranged to be met by Dottie Channing-Williams, the good natured landlady of a cosy racing pub, the Five Bells, just a few miles between the training centre at Lambourn and Bob's own home. Dottie—a warm, friendly person with a sharp sense of humour—had become a confidante of several of her customers. She readily offered help and sound advice to anyone with problems and, Bob had reasoned, there were worse ways of spending an evening than chatting to her beautiful twin daughters Karen and Nicole as they busied themselves around the pub and restaurant.

Dottie recalls the day she collected Bob at Heathrow. "He looked dreadful, tired and worried, but refused to tell me what was wrong until we arrived at his home. When we did get there he walked upstairs to have a bath. Only then would he talk seriously."

"Okay. If you must know," he revealed, "one of my balls is hard and swollen."

"Then you must do something about it. You must see a doctor," Dottie said.

"That's why I've come home."

Bob spent the next day, Sunday, at the Wickham charity horse show organized by Dottie Channing-Williams. He seemed unusually subdued but perked up when he met an attractive red-haired girl, Sally. They spent the evening together at the Five Bells and on Monday morning Bob, who was still banned from driving, was given a lift to the International Horse Show at Wembley where his great friend Derek Thompson was commentating for BBC radio. Bob met Derek for lunch, had a quick drink with him, then found a call box and rang Dr Alun Thomas at his Park Street surgery. When Alun Thomas came on the line Bob explained about the swelling and asked for an appointment as soon as possible.

"I can do better than that," replied Alun. "Give me your number and I'll call you there within ten minutes." Bob waited anxiously by the telephone.

Soon Alun Thomas rang back. He had fixed an appointment for Bob with a specialist at a hospital in the Fulham Road, Chelsea later in the afternoon. Bob made his way to the hospital, and after a lengthy examination the specialist asked him to return an hour later as he wanted a second opinion.

"The specialist had a look at everything and didn't seem very concerned so I wandered off to do some shopping," Bob recalls.

The decision of the two specialists after the second examination left Bob in a state of panic.

Although it didn't sink in at the time they told me they thought I had a tumour and they wanted me to enter hospital the very next day. I think they explained that they would operate, have a look and if they had to remove one of my balls then they would be able to recognize the type of tumour. I was told to go home and bring back my things the following day. The word cancer wasn't used that time but as I walked out I noticed the name of the hospital, the Royal Marsden, and suddenly remembered that was where Nicky, the girl I had met in Mexico, had been working. It was a cancer hospital.

When I twigged that I was petrified. I walked around London for two hours in a daze and didn't know where I was. I couldn't understand how I could be ill enough to need an operation when I felt so well. I didn't fancy any doctor operating on my balls. They are a very important part of a man's body.

Eventually Bob found a taxi to take him back to Wembley. There, while Derek was working, Bob started to drink on his own. He had arranged to stay in a spare bed in Derek's room on the top floor of the Crest Hotel. Midway through the evening he took the lift upstairs intending to shower and change his clothes. He brooded dejectedly as he paced alone in the hotel bedroom.

For the first time in my life I realized that I might die and so I decided to end it there and then. I rang my sister Mary and told her I was going to commit suicide. You don't hear about too many people recovering from cancer and that seemed the quickest way out. I thought I would jump out of the window but every time I looked out and saw how far it was to the ground I changed my mind. I was still in a state of shock.

The critical moment passed. Tortured with doubt about something he could not see and did not understand Bob returned to the bar and met Derek. The two friends sat discussing the problem late into the night.

"He told me he had quite seriously considered suicide by jumping out of the window," Derek says. "He calmed down a little as we talked. He's not a drinker but this time he was almost paralytic. When we went to bed at midnight he paced the floor for an hour or so muttering to himself, then disappeared off to the hotel nightclub looking for a girl. He was back ten minutes later on his own."

The next morning, Tuesday, 24th July, Bob returned home, packed a bag, caught a train to London and arrived back at the Royal Marsden Hospital just before lunch. There followed an endless series of tests.

> They must have taken eighteen or twenty different tests. They never stopped taking X-rays, making examinations, sticking needles into me and taking samples. I felt just like a pin cushion.

Sleep was impossible that night. Worried about his operation in the morning, anxious about his career and frightened about his very life, Bob was in a turmoil. During the pre-medical before the operation he panicked. Terrified by the implications he argued with the doctors and nurses until he drifted into unconsciousness.

> It was a horrible moment. I was going under not knowing if I was going to come out with one ball, two balls, or even, God help me, with none at all. When I woke up I thought they had been at work in the wrong place. They had opened me up several inches further up my tummy.

Bob soon learned that the surgeon had removed one testicle during the operation. This, it was hastily explained to him, would not interfere with his activities in any way. Tests were to be taken to discover if the tumour in the testicle that had been taken away was malignant.

One of Bob's first priorities was to ring Josh Gifford.

"How are you?" asked the trainer, who did not know his jockey had returned to England.

"Not brilliant," replied Bob. "I'll have to miss the first few days of the season as I'm in hospital."

"What's the matter? Have they gelded you at last? They should have done it a long time ago," laughed Josh.

"As a matter of fact they just have. I've just had the operation."

There was a ghastly silence on the phone. Poor Josh Gifford, completely unaware of the unfolding drama, was speechless as Bob explained the background to his operation.

A stream of visitors noted that the patient looked remarkably well. Always an impatient, restless character he badgered the hospital staff ceaselessly to allow him home and finally, after a few days, they succumbed to the pressure. First, however, he was sent as an out-patient for further tests to a second branch of the Royal Marsden Hospital at Sutton on the outskirts of London. There were more injections, X-rays, examinations and yet more tests including a kidney test and a body scan.

It was explained that he might need a course of radiation, so he was measured in case this was necessary. In addition dye was injected into the veins in the arches of his feet. This was uncomfortable rather than painful, and the resulting X-rays helped detect if the glands in his abdomen were normal and so unaffected. He still felt extraordinarily well though his morale was lowered by the incessant tests. But he wasn't particularly worried at this point.

I was still a bit sore from the operation, but there was no pain, so I tried it all out the following week and just as they had promised me everything still seemed to work normally. I imagined that was the end of my trouble though I realized I might have to have a course of radiation treatment.

Thirteen days after his operation he was called to London to meet the doctors again. They explained that the tests on the testicle that had been removed showed it had been malignant. His doctors believed the kick from Fury Boy had not caused his illness. More likely it had been a painful way of drawing attention to the disease already in his body. In medical terms he had a malignant teratoma. Worse, chest X-rays had revealed a shadow, or mass. The doctors wanted to operate again the following day to identify exactly the causes of that mass. Once more Bob argued, dismissing the shadow on the X-rays as no more significant than a scar from an old chest injury caused by a kick. He didn't want another operation. He felt so well, he was ready to resume riding and was already unhappy at missing the first week of the new season.

The unusual aspect about Bob's illness was that exhaustive tests did not find any evidence of glandular enlargement in his abdomen. Normally the spread from the testicles is into the lymph nodes near the kidneys and then steadily upwards as it expands into the chest. But tests did not detect anything wrong in his abdomen. Just to be absolutely sure, because the treatment was so drastic, the doctors wanted to take away a bit of a lymph node in his chest to confirm their fears that it was malignant. They explained carefully that it would be extremely useful if they could examine a part of the suspected tumour from his chest as well as the original tumour in one of his testicles. The operation would involve the removal of part of a rib to allow access to the mass in the centre of the chest.

Reluctantly, almost grudgingly, Bob agreed to the operation. Once more he returned home, packed his bags and was driven to hospital in London. When he arrived, there was an acute shortage of spare beds so at first he was put in a ward containing six old, extremely ill men, some who seemed close to death. That frightened Bob considerably and those of us who had accompanied him to the hospital left in a mood of dark despair. He was moved to another, brighter ward later that evening.

Bob's second operation was on Wednesday, 8th August. He woke up back in the ward with tubes coming out of his chest and a pump sucking excess fluid out, a painful process that continued for the next twelve hours. Cards, letters and flowers surrounded his bed and a bevy of dewy-eyed girls called to see him in relays but he was still too drowsy to pay them his usual alert attention. His first visitors included his parents, who lived near Lingfield racecourse, and his sister Mary. All the doubts, bitterness and resentment at the events of the previous few weeks overflowed into recrimination against his own family.

Says Mary, "Bob was really nasty. He shouted at Mum and me and snapped our heads off. He took it out on us and was horrible. He was just like a frightened, cornered animal and nothing we could do or say could ease his torment."

A welcome visitor the next evening was Josh Gifford with one of his younger owners, Henry Pelham.

"Josh brought me a large bottle of brandy," Bob recalls, "and with a bit of help from Henry drank most of it at one sitting."

Aware that Bob was convinced he would import another jockey Josh had hurried to the hospital to dispel those doubts. "I know racing's a cruel game, but I couldn't have been as cruel as to drop

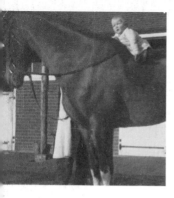

Bob Champion's first
rides: left at one year old;
centre at three, and
below Bob aged 10, with
Howard Thompson on
the pony behind and
Derek Thompson on
foot.

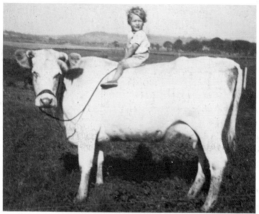

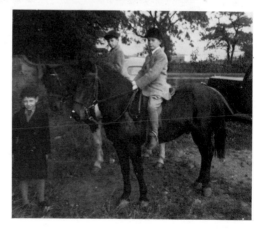

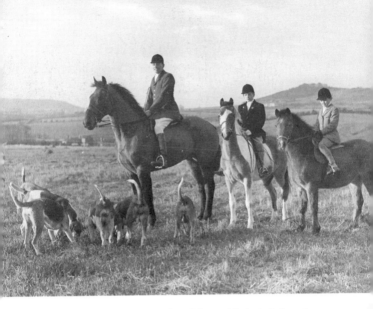

Bob aged 11 and his sister Mary with their father, then huntsman with the Cleveland.

Bob (*left*) aged 15 wins his first point-to-point.

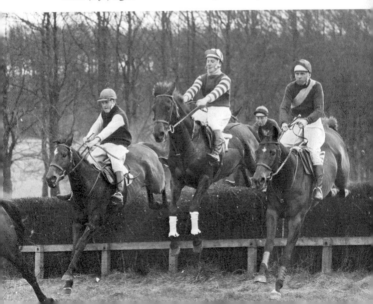

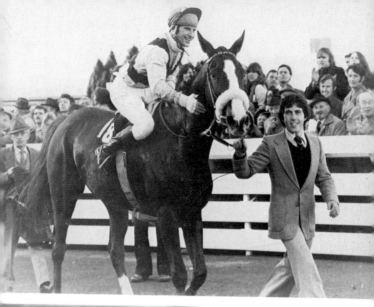

In the winners' enclosure after his finest victory to date – the 1978 Hennessy Cognac Gold Cup on Approaching.

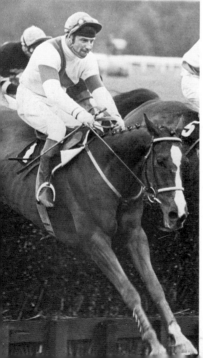

Bob and Aldaniti on their way to victory at Haydock in May 1979, two months before Bob learned he had cancer.

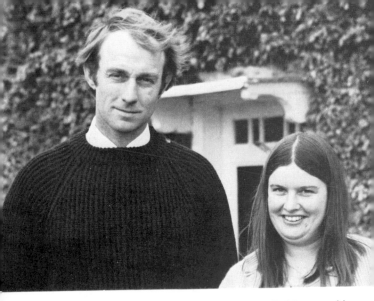

Richard and Mary Hussey who looked after Bob between his courses of chemotherapy.

Carol and Jenny, the sister and nurse at the Royal Marsden Hospital.

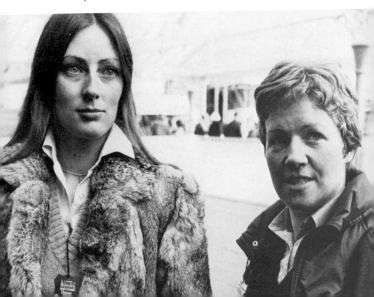

Bob, especially as we had enjoyed several really good seasons together."

Between sips of brandy Josh told Bob his job would be waiting, however long he took to recover. No-one could have known then how important that promise would become.

It was a tremendous incentive. He said it and I knew he meant it. He's always been a man of his word. Josh was absolutely terrific. If I'd lost the job I'd have given up. He gave me something to aim at, a spark of hope. That made all that followed easier for me to bear.

The following day Bob was deeply depressed—by his own circumstances, the smell of the hospital and the enclosed spaces of the ward. Allowed out of bed for the first time, he slipped on his dressing-gown and slippers, wandered aimlessly along endless corridors, through the front door, kept walking and found himself in a busy London street on a warm, sunny morning. Unaware of the surprised glances at his state of dress, he peered through shop windows, relishing in his new found freedom and eventually, reluctantly, made his way back to his ward where he was met by an irate doctor and a clutch of worried nurses.

The doctor gave me a right bollocking. One of the nurses had seen me in the street and they were in a state of alarm. The doctor said if I wanted to go anywhere I must have a nurse with me.

He said they had a responsibility to look after me and the least I could do if I wished to recover was to co-operate. He made it clear that if I was going to behave like a child I might just as well go home the following day. So, being in an awkward mood, I did. At that stage I was past caring. I felt they were just using me as a guinea-pig and I'd had enough. All I wanted to do was start riding again and that seemed less and less possible.

Chapter 6

AFTER A MISERABLE weekend at home Bob was driven to the Royal Marsden Hospital at Sutton on Monday, 13th August by his long-suffering girl friend Sally. They had known each other for less than a month but already she had become involved in a situation that would have tested the devotion, patience and endurance of a woman twice her age. The journey to hospital that morning was not a happy one.

"His temper was dreadful," Sally says. "He kept shouting 'Move into this lane or that lane' and that I was doing it all wrong. I told him to shut up but still he kept on at me. He was impossible and kept saying he knew the quickest way, all the short cuts and that I had taken the wrong road. Finally I'd had enough. I pulled in by the side of the road, jumped out of the car and told him to get on with it. He just looked at me in the embarrassed way he does and very quietly apologized. That shows how upset he was because normally he never apologizes."

They reached Sutton in time for Bob's appointment with his doctors. All weekend he had been worrying about his illness. Now, at last, he would learn the truth. Sitting uneasily in a small room at the hospital, his heart pounding, he listened as if in a dream as the two doctors explained he had cancer and only eight months or so to live unless he was prepared to try an immediate, drastic course of chemotherapy treatment. He argued and resisted that harsh verdict and doubted if he was being told the truth. Finally, inevitably, he relented, accepted the doctors' diagnosis and agreed to begin the first course of treatment that very day.

The next four hours were the most traumatic of Bob Champion's life. It was explained that one of several nasty side effects of the treatment would almost certainly leave him sterile. That news would shatter any man, but to someone like Bob—who loved children, was godfather to several and had always looked forward to having his own children when he married—it was a desperate blow. At once he was sent to the sperm bank in the hospital. There sperm samples produced by patients can be stored for several years at the correct temperature, but Bob, to his eternal regret, was unable to leave an effective specimen.

The sample I gave was not good enough. The drugs and effects of the two operations had shaken up my system. I was told I would have to wait a few weeks for everything in my body to settle down before I could give a reliable sample. But I didn't have the time to spare. I had to get on with the treatment immediately. I was in such a state that I wasn't sure I'd be around afterwards and there seemed little point in leaving something in a sperm bank. Basically I didn't have a proper chance to leave a specimen. I couldn't afford to wait for days, let alone the number of weeks they suggested.

More tests followed, then an administrative muddle sent Bob to the wrong ward—an acute medical division full mostly of seriously ill old men confined to bed. Bob sat in the corridor of the ward for two, perhaps three, hours in a state of panic. Several times he wandered to the call-box at the end of the ward to ring friends; for the rest of the time he gripped Sally's hand tightly.

I was waiting to see the ward doctor and was so frightened by what I saw that I decided I definitely wasn't staying. The fear of the unknown is the greatest fear of all. I still didn't know what I had let myself in for but the sight of all those people in the ward put the fear of God up me. None of them looked as if they would last long. My mind was made up that I was going and Sally had to restrain me two or three times from walking out. As I was leaving someone at last realized the mistake and directed me to the right ward.

So Sally led him upstairs to the Pinkham ward on the third floor. There they waited nervously once more. Sally remembers the day vividly.

"We didn't have to wait long this time but it was still awful. Old men and young lads wandered around, all of them completely bald. It was the first time Bob had actually seen what he had to face. One lad came past with a huge operation scar on his chest. He was carrying a metal stanchion and there were various tubes attached to his body."

At last a friendly sister, tall, dark and briskly efficient, called out, "Bob, what on earth are you doing here?" It was Nicky, the nursing sister he had met on holiday in Mexico two months earlier while she had been on an exchange course. The knowledge that someone he knew was in charge of the ward was a brief, welcome relief, but, alarmed by the sight of so many people so obviously ill, Bob insisted on being given a single, private room. That demand would not normally have been considered, let alone granted, but luckily a patient who had been using the only male private room in the ward was in the process of being transferred. The bed was available.

Sally comments, "Bob created a right disturbance and wouldn't calm down until he was sure he had his own room. Really he was like a little boy. He behaved like that because he was so frightened."

At first one of the nurses, Jenny, sat down with him to check his medical history. That informal chat is a practical and sensible way of breaking the ice between nurses and new patients. It helps calm the patient and establish mutual trust. Later the ward doctor did exactly the same thing and then explained how the chemotherapy would be administered. Before being put to bed Bob was sent for a kidney function test, an injection of fluid that measures the amount of blood flowing through the kidneys. Correct kidney function is vital for patients who are given a liquid platinum compound as part of the chemotherapy treatment. Platinum is toxic (poisonous) and can cause kidney failure, so for much of the five days of each course patients are given continuous fluids to flush their kidneys through. Later in the afternoon when the results of the tests were known, one of the nurses implanted a cannula, a permanent hollow tube that enters a vein in the arm and is used as a funnel to administer intravenous treatment. Each cannula is supposed to last the full five days of a course of treatment but in practice they don't usually survive more than two or three days.

That first Monday, 13th August, was to be day 0 of the first of six treatments for Bob Champion. At ten o'clock in the evening the duty nurse put him on the first of numerous drips, a normal saline solution, a mixture of salt and water. She hung the bag on a stanchion by his bedside and connected it to the cannula in his arm.

It was awkward rather than uncomfortable and at first was just a nuisance. You are aware of the liquid dripping into your system all the while and so it's difficult to rest or sleep. Everywhere I moved, around the ward or to the bathroom, I had to take the stanchion carrying the bag. That first night I didn't sleep partly because of the discomfort and partly because I was so terrified.

At ten o'clock on Tuesday morning, day 1, the saline drip was exchanged for twenty minutes or so by a much smaller bag containing liquid platinum, the first of the three drugs used to treat Bob's particular type of cancer. This was followed by an intravenous injection of a second drug, vinblastine. Then the saline drip was re-connected. That first day Bob managed to eat a little of the hospital breakfast but later he couldn't face lunch or supper and for the rest of his stays in hospital didn't even bother to inspect the menu to order any meals. "I felt sick, and the very sight or smell of food only made me worse," he says.

He would sip a little Coca Cola or Tizer, sometimes a mouthful of weak tea, but solid food was out of the question. His weight dropped dramatically during that first six-day spell in hospital.

On day 2, platinum, vinblastine and the third drug, bleomycin were all administered through his cannula. That night he began to vomit for the first time.

It annoyed me at first. Remember I had felt so well until going into hospital and I was convinced they were experimenting on me, using me solely as a guinea-pig. I still sometimes wonder now. How could you be made to be so ill only days after feeling so well?

On Thursday, day 3, platinum alone was administered between bouts of the saline solution. Many visitors had called to see Bob who, understandably, had never felt less like being sociable. A constant worry was the rotation of his dozen or so heartbroken girlfriends so that any two of them should not meet, let alone clash, sad-eyed at his bedside.

A second major worry was finance. As a self-employed jockey Bob's income when he was ill or injured was negligible. He did not qualify for the usual grants from the Racecourse Compensation Fund and his sole income during his entire illness was the usual £14.70 weekly sickness benefit. His insurance proved worthless as his type of illness was ruled out in the small print. The Injured Jockeys Fund, a registered charity, stepped in at once with substantial support that eased his anxiety and paid outstanding bills. Two of the Fund's trustees Lord John Oaksey and Brough Scott had both ridden against Bob and were concerned that financial matters should not be a worry at all during his illness. They arranged for the Fund to help with a considerable loan paid direct to his accountant, who was then able to attend to the usual bills. The Fund, in short, settled some of his immediate commitments and removed the problem of money from his mind for the time being. The costs of his previous treatment, including the two operations, came close to three thousand pounds. Some of it was met by BUPA, the rest by the Injured Jockeys Fund.

On day 4 Bob felt increasingly ill. He ate nothing and spent hours staring at his portable television without taking any notice. On day 5, Friday, there were further infusions of platinum.

The nurses and sisters, who took such pains to encourage Bob, explained that he had a stage three testicular tumour, something that tended to occur in men between the ages of twenty and forty. Although the incidence was only about two per cent of all cancers, it was the second most common cancer in young men. Had the tumour been diagnosed earlier, perhaps while he was in America, he might well have needed radiation treatment only. Once Bob understood the implications of his illness he was better prepared to face the treatment to cure it.

Tumour cells, he was told, grew faster than ordinary cells. A teratoma, the growth which was Bob's particular complaint, doubles in size every twenty to twenty-seven days. Malignant cells divide more rapidly than normal cells. Chemotherapy is the most effective way so far invented of attacking the evil spread of the rapidly dividing cells. Normal circulation ensures that the toxic drugs reach every single cell in a patient's body and kill off the rapidly dividing cells. Because the doubling time of the tumour is so fast the tumour also responds quickly to treatment.

Carol, the second of the two ward sisters and Jenny, a good-natured, practical nurse spent much time reassuring the new patient. "Bob was quite anxious that first week and asked a lot of questions," says Carol, "but that was quite good because at least he voiced his fears rather than bottling them up inside. In a way he was a better person because he expressed his doubts. He wanted to know everything. Because he told us what was frightening him we were able to help him. The most difficult patients are the ones who keep their fears to themselves.

"Each patient reacts differently. You can warn them of some of the more unpleasant side effects but the main thing they all knew was that if they were worried about anything while away from hospital they could call us at any time. The patients are encouraged to ring us as well as their doctors. We know from experience of other patients what kind of harmful effects these drugs cause whereas the average doctor may not have come across some of the drugs."

Before he left hospital at the end of the first of what he hoped would be four courses of treatment, Bob was warned that he would suffer from constipation. More serious, he learned that his resistance to infection would be considerably and dangerously lowered within a few days and he was given a letter to show to his local doctor in case of emergency. There was a very real risk of becoming perilously ill with septicaemia.

On day 6, Saturday, 18th August, he was driven home by Sally. On the way they stopped at the Five Bells where Bob, to his surprise, was able to eat a steak and salad. At the best of times Bob is a stubborn, independent person. Now, despite much advice to the contrary, he was determined to continue living at home by himself—given, of course, the usual visits from his various girlfriends. On Sunday he had been hoping to travel down to Dorset to make an appearance at Jim Old's annual charity cricket match, but by mid-morning he began to feel very ill. He retired to bed, moaning in constant pain, and Sally became so worried by his

71

condition later in the day that she asked Dottie Channing-Williams to visit him. Dottie has a vivid memory of that visit: "Bob was lying under the bedcovers groaning, 'Who's there? Help me, help me.' But he didn't want us to call the doctor."

Bob was unable to sleep. Sweating profusely he began to vomit and suffered from the most agonizing stomach cramp. Weak and light-headed he struggled, exhausted, through the night and soon after five on Monday morning rang his sister Mary Hussey, and begged her to collect him. Richard Hussey, a big, practical man, drove the twenty miles or so to Bob's home and was shocked by his brother-in-law's appearance. "It was obvious he was very ill. He was rough. He had acute stomach ache, felt sick and was in terrible pain."

By nine that morning Bob was tucked up safely in the spare bedroom at the Hussey's farmhouse a mile from the market town of Wootton Bassett. His condition deteriorated. Just as he had been warned by the doctors he suffered the most agonizing constipation. Milpar, a vile tasting white liquid given to him to ease the condition, made no difference. In desperation he took some of his old laxative pills that he had previously used to lose weight quickly when he was riding. Normally their effect on his system was drastic and immediate, but now even they failed to ease the blockage.

Mary was deeply concerned by Bob's condition and called out her local doctor three days running. She recalls: "Bob had been warned he would be bad but this was worse than anything you could imagine. I used to stay up all night with him. He'd be in bed all the time and when he tried to get up to go to the bathroom he kept falling over. I didn't know how we were going to manage for six months like that. The thing that crossed both our minds was that he might die here in the house. We didn't know then whether he was going to live or not."

On Wednesday, 22nd August, day 9 of the first course of treatment, Richard drove Bob back to the hospital in Sutton where he was given his scheduled injection of bleomycin after the customary blood test. He was also given an enema to help end the constipation, but that too failed to work. After two hours at the hospital Richard drove him back to the farm.

By now messages and phone calls from various girlfriends had begun to filter through. "They were all a bloody nuisance," says Mary. "He didn't want to talk to them or see them. They were a pain in the neck for him and us. In the end we told them to stop calling. Some of them were so persistent and extremely rude."

Richard laughs. "In fairness to them they all thought they were *the* special one and couldn't understand why we were protecting him." He pauses, then adds drily, "There must have been thirty special ones! They never really stopped ringing then and they haven't now."

Bob's young niece, Emma, aged seven at the time, proved a gentle, thoughtful nurse. She would tiptoe into his room, bring what he wanted and generally make a fuss of him. Her brother, Nicky, aged six, worried about his Uncle Bob and would pop up to his room too, every so often, to see that he was all right. Bob's acute state of constipation had become a matter of concern for everyone at the farm. The first question asked in the morning would centre on his activities in the bathroom. One morning Richard was working in a field near the house when Nicky came running towards him shouting urgently.

"I thought something terrible had happened until I could see Nick was laughing," says Richard. "Then I heard him shouting happily, 'Dad, Dad, Uncle Bobby's been!' "

The constipation, however, was not a joke for the sufferer.

It was worse than you can imagine. I'd sit on the throne for half an hour at a time reading the *Sporting Life* just praying something would happen. I'd try my heart out. The sweat would pour off me, but nothing would happen. I was also sick a lot because I was still constipated and so there was nowhere else for the food to go. It would come straight back up again ten minutes after every meal. I tried all sorts of recommended aids to end the constipation but nothing succeeded. My bowels were simply not working. The worst time was the first treatment. I didn't go for seventeen days, but after I'd been once I could always go again.

As predicted, too, towards the end of the first cycle of twenty-one days his hair began to fall out, at first just the odd wisp, but soon in larger tufts.

I had persuaded myself it wouldn't happen and so it was quite a shock to wake up in the mornings and find bits of my hair all over the pillow.

Wild rumours began to sweep racecourses about Bob's illness. His absence from the start of the season had been noted despite lack of comment in the newspapers. The nature of his illness became known and at the Brighton meeting on 22nd August the story quickly spread that he had died. The *Sporting Life* even prepared a front-page obituary with a suitable photograph from their picture library, but a few check calls soon put an end to that dismal tale before it was printed. A great friend, Terry Biddlecombe, was so upset at hearing the news of Bob's death that he rang the Husseys to check its validity. Bob answered the phone.

"You can cancel the wreath," he told Terry.

Others, too, rang with the same morbid question so Bob determined on a foolish plan to end the rumours. Although barely fit to walk around the house in his dressing-gown he arranged for Bob Davies to take him to the next Fontwell meeting on 29th August, which happened to be day 16 of the treatment. He was due that day at hospital for a further injection of bleomycin but, typically, put that off for twenty-four hours.

I wanted to show everyone I was all right and Fontwell was the ideal place. It was a stupid thing to do but I was mad. How would you feel if people kept saying you were supposed to be dead? I wanted to make a show but nearly killed myself doing it. Even so that was the first time I really started fighting. It irritated me more than anything.

Bob Davies, three-times champion jockey, picked his friend up early in the morning and they drove to Josh Gifford's stables at Findon for lunch before racing. Later they moved on to Fontwell where Bob was so weak and cold that he hid for most of the afternoon in the warmth of the weighing-room. He looked so pale, thin and ill that many of his friends, appalled at his appearance, feared the rumours might soon become fact.

Bob returned to the farm exhausted, but the following day was driven by Richard Hussey back to the hospital at Sutton for his latest injection of bleomycin. In the final week of the cycle he began to feel much better. He started to eat more food and, wearing dressing-gown and slippers, would come down to the farmhouse kitchen and sit on a chair with his feet resting on top of the huge Aga while the open oven door kept him warm. At last he felt well enough to use the telephone and so rang all his friends outlining his progress. In the evenings he would stay downstairs in front of a roaring log fire spending hours on the phone while Richard and Mary, like so many farming families, retired early to bed. Nick and Emma soon nicknamed him "Tinkle, Tinkle Bob" because he was always on the telephone.

When Bob collected his car, which had been sitting idle outside the Five Bells for three weeks, it wouldn't start and a mechanic from the local garage discovered that sugar had been put in the petrol tank. The tank had to be drained and cleaned. Bob borrowed Richard's car and drove thirty miles to visit Arthur and Eileen Corp, the relatives who had helped start his riding career in point-to-points. He also spent an enjoyable two days with Bob and Sue Davies whose youngest child Nick is one of his godchildren.

By now his hair was coming out in chunks but on Sunday, 2nd September he insisted on attending the Christening party for Katie Powell. On his arm was an attractive redhead, Corinne. The day was sunny and warm but Bob, noticeably, felt cold and stayed indoors most of the afternoon. Those people who had not seen him for some time felt he looked desperately ill. No wonder they found it hard to accept his entirely accurate explanation that the harsh treatment rather than the illness itself was the cause of his gaunt, listless appearance.

Chapter 7

BOB RETURNED TO the Royal Marsden hospital at Sutton on Monday, 3rd September to start his second cycle of treatment. He sat subdued and silent in the car as Richard drove steadily through the Monday morning rush-hour traffic around London.

> By then I knew what to expect. They had told me it would be much worse the second time. I was petrified at the prospect of going back.

This time even his considerable charm was unable to persuade the nurses to give him a private room again as it was already taken, so, after the usual tests, he moved into a small room with six beds, some of them occupied. After he had been re-connected to the saline drip there was time to contemplate the sorry state of his hair.

He had finally accepted his hair would fall out because he'd seen it happen to all the others in the ward. On the first morning back in hospital he woke up with bits of hair in his face, eyes and ears, so reluctantly agreed that one of the nurses should shave the rest of it off. Edna, a friendly Chinese nurse, was the girl chosen to perform this depressing task. Wielding a cut-throat razor with practised skill, she scythed off the remaining hair on his head. His sideboards, too, had begun to fall out so Edna shaved those off as well. When she had finished only his eyebrows remained. Anxiously he asked for a mirror and stared morosely at the unknown skinhead who confronted him.

> I looked terrible. Like a man from another planet. I hated losing my hair. I'm extremely vain, you know. I think it affected my whole personality. My head felt cold, different, and I was defenceless.

Relief was at hand. Patients are allowed two wigs, supplied by the hospital and can choose from a variety of styles, colours and lengths. Bob picked out two that he felt would suit him and enjoyed the next stage as the hospital hairdresser trimmed them to his specification. Somehow Bob ended up with four wigs after the supplier believed his unlikely story that a horse had eaten one. He kept them on the four bedposts in his room.

I had one for best, one for going out in, one for sleeping in and one I wore around the farm.

At the hospital, when he was among others with the same problem, Bob didn't bother to wear a wig, but when he was staying with Richard and Mary or going out he would always wear one.

"At that stage," he insists, "I didn't give a damn about women." Even so he always donned a wig when he was expecting yet another female visitor.

That second spell in hospital was quite appalling. Once the chemotherapy treatment started again Bob vomited constantly, often as much as ten or twelve times in an hour. He could not face any food, sipped only a little liquid and for much of the day lay groaning in bed.

Soon I was being sick and there was nothing to come up. I'd lie there feeling weaker and weaker and every so often would retch and heave. One man being sick in the ward would start the others off. It was so bad that every time Steph, the prettiest nurse, came in I was sick.

Night brought little respite. Bob would try to sleep but managed only the odd hour's cat-nap. He felt desperately ill and at times his ambition to ride Aldaniti in the Grand National the following spring seemed an absurd, impossible dream. "The way I felt most of the time I couldn't have ridden a bicycle."

As he lay sick and dispirited, numerous gifts arrived by his bedside.

Champagne, chocolates, cigars, cakes, biscuits, whisky, sweets, all the things I couldn't face.

Bob was much sicker than the average patient on chemotherapy, perhaps because he had been so much fitter when he started the treatment. He would lie for hours staring miserably at the ceiling and became so depressed and grumpy that the nurses clubbed together to buy him a "happy" hat. He did not appreciate the joke. Sometimes he would watch racing on his portable television, but that depressed him even more because Josh Gifford was having such a wonderful run and he knew he was missing so many winners. Josh would pop in to see him whenever he could and privately doubted that Bob would ride again. A great friend of his, Alan Oughton, who also trained at Findon, had died from cancer a few years earlier and Josh could remember the same encouraging noises before Alan's death.

"Oh no," says Josh. "I definitely didn't think Bob would ride again though I made sure it was not obvious when I talked to him. When he was on the treatment it was horrible to see. It made you ill just to go in there. I dreaded it. I mean I honestly didn't think he would ever come out of the hospital. I don't know much about medicine but owners of mine who seemed to be aware of the full implications of his illness, including one who lives next door to the hospital, gave me the impression that Bob had no chance of surviving. But Bob's sister Mary was always confident when I spoke to her and that gave me a bit of hope."

Another frequent caller was Josh's efficient secretary Judy Bradley, sister of the showjumper Caroline Bradley. She would always bring presents and messages from friends at the stable. Judy recalls, "Whenever the doctors gave him good news he would ask quite seriously 'Can I cancel the undertaker?' "

Bob's most regular visitors were his mother, Frank Pullen and Monty Court. Frank Pullen and his father, builders from south London, had always had a horse or two with Josh Gifford and had formed a close friendship with the stable jockey. Bob had won on several of the Pullens' horses including Charlotson and Man on the Moon. Frank, a chatty cockney, lived forty miles away in Sevenoaks, often worked in London and visited Bob every day that he was in hospital.

"In all the time Bob was riding for myself and dad," Frank says, "he was always open and honest about our horses. He's completely straightforward. He told us the truth about our horses even if we didn't want to hear it and we became good mates.

"Most of the time in hospital he just talked about riding again and the Grand National. At other times he would be asleep and so I'd creep away without waking him. Often he was too ill to talk. To me he was a million dollars. One day he made me go with him while he had a series of injections. It made me ill just to watch."

Monty Court, the racing editor of the *Sunday Mirror*, lived a few miles away from the hospital and tried to call most days. If it was in the morning he would bring a *Sporting Life*, racing's Bible, and a bottle or two of soft drinks; if it was in the evening he would provide another newspaper and a bag of plums or grapes. Monty remembers the unusually high degree of heating in the Pinkham ward. "It was hot, even by hospital standards; once when I arrived I found Bob sitting outside on the roof cooling down. I did my best to jolly him along but he wasn't in a very funny mood. He didn't talk much. All he wanted was something to sweeten his mouth to take away the taste of vomit. My idea was to visit often and briefly. Once I asked what the food was like. He looked at me as if I'd asked a daft question, then croaked, 'I don't know.' He'd go days without eating anything except the odd piece of fruit. There was a time, too, when he'd done something rather silly and the duty nurse gave him a fierce rollocking. She knew how to handle him and he took it in the right spirit."

Much of the time Bob was too ill for even the most banal chatter. The ward sister Carol reveals, "I'm sure he felt we were not telling him everything. He imagined it was a huge conspiracy by the hospital to use him as a suitable guinea-pig for the new treatment. At first he kept asking and asking, seeking re-assurance. We had to show him X-rays and the results of all his tests. He had to see everything written down.

"Even when we gave him good news, such as when the X-rays showed the tumour in his chest was regressing, he would demand to see for himself. He had to see everything in black and white. It was not perhaps so much that he didn't believe us, more that he wanted solid evidence of his progress. He felt so ill he couldn't believe he was improving."

The dosage of the three drugs, platinum, vinblastine and bleomycin, is calculated according to the body size of each patient. The seriousness of the chemotherapy treatment in a twenty-one day cycle may best be shown by listing the various side effects caused by the three main drugs.

Platinum led to severe nausea and vomiting, anorexia, bone marrow depression—which stops the production of blood cells—and pins and needles. Vinblastine also caused anorexia, loss of weight and appetite, pins and needles and bone marrow depression. Bleomycin was responsible for baldness, constipation, pigmentation of skin—especially on the back of the neck, on scars and scratch marks—mild bone marrow depression, severe cramping pain as a result of tumour breakdown and mouth ulcers.

No wonder Bob claims, "In killing off the cancer the drugs just about kill you as well in the process."

Various antidotes, pills and injections were used to reduce some of the side effects. Largactil, prescribed as an anti-sickness drug, was given in tablet form but Bob would be sick at the very sight of them so eventually the nurses gave him Largactil in a saline drip which lasted half an hour. Its main purpose was to make a patient drowsy but for some reason it did not have the same effect on him as on others. Maxalon, another anti-sickness drug also failed to cure his constant vomiting. As for Milpar, the vile tasting liquid taken to ease constipation, Bob adamantly refused to take the stuff.

John Gobourn, who runs his own garage and plant hire business near Aberystwyth, had started the treatment at the same time as Bob. The pair became good friends though they were too ill to converse for much of the time. John, who suffered from the same type of cancer as Bob, had been given only three months to live in 1978 by specialists at a Welsh hospital and was then treated by radiation. It worked for a while but when the cancer began to spread again John asked for a second opinion and had been sent to the Royal Marsden.

"There are no words that can adequately describe how awful having the chemotherapy treatment could be," John says. "I was horribly sick and I was quite lucky. Bob had a much tougher time than me. However bad he was, his only thought was to get back riding and we each worked out to the exact hour how long we would be stuck in hospital."

After six days Bob was ready to be taken back to the Hussey's farm (there was no question this time of him returning to his own house), but first he insisted on a piping hot bath. He explains.

You could always smell the platinum on your body. It was horrible. I would wake up and stink of it, especially if I had been sweating. You couldn't have a bath while you were on the drip so the end of the course was an ideal time.

Unfortunately Bob was far too weak to cope with the steamy heat of a hot bath. His last-day bath, which became something of a ritual, usually ended abruptly when he collapsed, either in the bath or on the floor of the bathroom. Weightless and dizzy he would lie helplessly waiting to be rescued. The good-natured nurse Jenny, aware of the problem, would station herself near the door in readiness to pick him up.

When I drove him home on the evening of Saturday 8th September, he twice asked me to stop for a moment so that he could be sick. But as we sped down the M4 further towards Wiltshire his mood brightened perceptibly and by the time we reached Wootton Bassett he was ready for his first proper meal in a week. The excesses of the next two days soon ended as the dreaded constipation returned. Once more he was in acute pain with severe stomach cramps. Once more all the usual aids failed to end the blockage, but at least it didn't last so long as the first time. Again towards the end of the second week out of hospital he felt a marked improvement in his condition. He walked a little round the farm, called to see several friends in the area and resumed his favourite pastime on the telephone. He was also able to act as temporary telex operator by sending a series of messages on his brother-in-law's machine to Richard's business contacts in Saudi Arabia.

When he was well enough he would sit for hours in front of the roaring fire in the front room watching video films of his greatest triumphs. Everyone else in the house soon tired of the sight of Bob Champion winning the same races repeatedly but he was certainly cheered by the constant reminder of happier days. The very act of replaying the video tapes strengthened his resolve to ride again.

At that stage, Bob reasoned, he was halfway through the planned treatment. The hospital were pleased with his progress when he returned on the ninth and sixteenth days for injections. His blood tests were promising. X-rays showed the tumour in his chest had reduced considerably. He had, however, lost a tremendous amount of weight and barely touched nine stone on the scales; his face was the colour and texture of ancient, yellowing parchment. Nicky and Emma, amused by his bald head, quickly renamed him "Uncle Kojak".

For the first time in his life, Bob considered making a will.

I had little choice but to accept what had happened though there were times when I didn't think I would survive. I thought of writing a will but decided against it as that seemed to be tempting fate. I knew if I died all my insurance would go to mum and dad and really I wasn't sane enough at the time to make a will.

Judy Bradley or Josh Gifford would ring regularly with news of the stable and in particular Aldaniti, who was back in training after a lengthy rest in the summer. He was due to run towards the end of November and whatever his doctors thought Bob intended to be there to see the race.

By then I had an obsession about winning the Grand National on Aldaniti in March 1980. I would lie in bed night after night believing we would win and the thought of anyone else riding him was too painful to consider. He was my ride and I was going to be there to ride him. He made a perfect target for me to regain fitness. I had worked out that after the four treatments ended towards the end of October I still had five months to get fit before the National.

Aldaniti's owners, Nick and Valda Embiricos, and Josh Gifford hoped he might be back in time. "Oh yes," says Josh. "If Bob had been fit enough to ride Aldaniti in the Grand National he would have done so. Nick and Valda would have loved him to ride the horse. So would I."

Bob returned to hospital to start his third course of treatment on Monday, 24th September. His knowledge of what lay ahead in the next few days did not ease the pain and discomfort, but there was just one advantage of chemotherapy treatment. The hair on his face, as on every part of his body, had fallen out so he no longer had to shave in the morning.

Once more the chemotherapy caused him to be violently sick and he showed no interest at all in the hospital food. The only meal he would consider was rice pudding. On his return to hospital he brought with him several tins of rice pudding which were duly taken to the canteen and cooked to his specifications, and he lived for most of the week on that and orange juice. When the orange ran out one day he summoned Carol hastily. She was unable to leave the ward to find the precious liquid but called on Les, a hospital porter, who enjoyed nothing more in his spare time than backing horses.

When Bob was first admitted, Les, on seeing his name on the list, rang the Pinkham ward asking, "Is that *the* Bob Champion? I've won some money on him in the past. Anytime he wants something let me know."

Now the moment had come to repay that favour. No sooner had Carol asked him than Les sprinted across to the nearest shop, bought the orange juice and sent it as a matter of priority to the ward.

Bob's mother, Derek Thompson and Dottie Channing-Williams were frequent visitors. During the later cycles of treatment Derek would force himself to bully his great friend. He recalls, "Bob would be lying there in bed, being sick, feeling sorry for himself and I'd start on him. 'Have you been for a walk round the wards this morning? You must keep moving if you are going to ride again. You can't let your muscles waste away.' Bob would curse me then drag himself painfully and slowly out of bed and stumble round the room once or twice hanging on to the stanchion. Sometimes he couldn't get out of bed. He was simply too weak.

"Then a fortnight or so later he would ring to say he wanted a day at the races. He always tried to go once in between treatments. He'd walk around in the bitter cold looking like death. Sometimes I could see it was an effort for him to stand up but he usually had a girl to support him."

Presents and parcels continued to arrive at the hospital. The gifts normally contained food or books but Bob, like so many people in racing, is not a man who reads very much. The *Sporting Life*, *Playboy* magazine and racing form books are the sum total of his library at home.

"The last two things he wanted at the time were food and books," says Carol, the ward sister. "He couldn't eat and was too ill to read. After a while he was so low he would throw the parcels aside and not even open them for several days. He'd groan, 'Not another bloody Dick Francis novel.' By the time he left here he must have had several complete collections of Dick Francis novels and I don't think he looked at any of them. He gave several away."

The stream of female visitors had slowed to a trickle, though Jenny, a red-haired amateur rider, proved a constant support. Everyone on the ward was fascinated by his selection of girlfriends and by the way he charmed the switchboard operators at the hospital to allow him priority use of the phone. Carol takes up the story again: "There was a continuous flow of eighteen-year-olds to see him. The kind that walked in as if they owned the place. Most of the time he didn't want to see them and we had to make a lot of excuses for him. One girl asked us to give her a room for a few minutes so that she could put on her make-up and then told me to let her know when all the other visitors had gone because she didn't want to be seen with the rabble!"

Each five-day course of intensive chemotherapy left Bob weak, depressed and at times exhausted. The permanent flood of various fluids into his system became an endless, torturous nightmare. The chemotherapy, he knew, was the cause of his terrible sickness, and soon he persuaded the ward nurses and sisters to give him an hour's break from the treatment each morning at around ten o'clock. "He was never awkward but always insisted on his hour off," says Jenny, one of the nurses.

If the fluid had gone through a bit sooner than scheduled he felt that a break from the endless supply into his body could only do him good. He would wander around the wards, free at last from his regular companion, the stanchion. But the relief was only temporary.

I came to dread the sight of the drip in my arm all the time. At night it was impossible to sleep. Anti-sickness drugs didn't work on me and even the ones to make me drowsy were not very effective. I'd lie awake at night, wondering if I would ever walk out of the hospital again. One of the hardest things for me was that I was the first professional sportsman to have been there. No-one seemed very confident that I would ride again. They didn't seem to know, but were worried about my wind more than anything.

His doctor, Jane Merrow, had explained the possible harmful effects of the drug bleomycin. She feared it would cause a serious loss of lung volume or breathing capacity. The doctors were fully aware that bleomycin reduced lung function by a third, although some patients regained part of that by adjusting and exercising. Thus after the treatment they were left with only two-thirds of their original lung capacity, a percentage gauged accurately from a series of tests. Such a loss wouldn't matter for the average person in an ordinary job which didn't require a high degree of physical effort. Obviously it would make a crucial difference to Bob's effectiveness as a jockey, particularly towards the end of a race. But it was possible that pressure on his lungs from the mass of lymph glands had hampered his breathing in the final months before his illness was discovered. That, at least, would improve as the treatment caused the tumour to diminish.

Bob, who does not smoke cigarettes or cigars, brooded on the problem night after night until he left hospital on Saturday 29th September at the end of his third course of treatment. Once more he was reminded of the dangers of septicaemia. It was a timely warning, as events were to show.

Chapter 8

IN THE COURSE of six treatments of chemotherapy the majority of patients with Bob's particular type of cancer return to the hospital at one time or another with blood poisoning. Septicaemia occurs when a patient's blood count and resistance to infection is at its lowest, usually around the ninth and tenth days of each cycle. Those who live a long way from the hospital are not allowed out until the critical period has passed and they are no longer in danger. The risk of death from blood poisoning is a very real one. The complications from a simple cold can kill if not treated with massive doses of the correct antibiotic. A few cancer patients out of the hundreds at the hospital have died from septicaemia. There is a two per cent mortality rate from side effects of the treatment, and Bob Champion came perilously close to adding to that grim statistic.

During the first week after the third treatment Bob stayed in bed at the farmhouse except for his brief return to the hospital on day 9, Wednesday 3rd October, for the usual tests and injections. As usual at that stage he was constipated, sick and depressed.

He did not think it was possible to feel any worse but when he woke up on Sunday 7th October he was aware of painful, unpleasant mouth sores. As the day progressed spots broke out on his face and neck and he started shivering and sweating. He felt feverish and eventually, in the afternoon, forced himself downstairs to tell Mary. He lay by the fire in his dressing-gown for a while, then grudgingly stood outside in a gateway for a few minutes while some loose cattle were rounded up. He was miserable, bad-tempered and shouted angrily at seven-year-old Emma. Richard was out on the farm planting wheat, and Mary suggested Bob returned to bed while she finished off the chain harrowing in another field. When she returned to the house she was alarmed at the deterioration in his condition: "He had gone downhill visibly," she says.

Just before six Mary phoned the hospital who advised her to take Bob's temperature. A frantic search failed to unearth a thermometer so Mary rang a friend, Briar Elliott, who rushed round with one. Bob's temperature was 102 degrees. Mary rang the hospital again, desperately worried by now, and she also called her own doctor to attend Bob as a matter of urgency.

He examined Bob and rang the hospital at Sutton as requested in the note Bob had kept from his first treatment. The advice was firm. Bob must go straight to hospital, either locally at Swindon or back to the hospital where he was being treated. The debate was a difficult one. Time was clearly critical and the drive back to the outskirts of London on Sunday night would take the best part of two hours. Mary's doctor, however, felt—quite correctly—that Bob's own hospital, though much further away, was much better equipped to understand and cope with the emergency.

Immediately the decision was taken Mary sent Nicky off in his pyjamas with a torch to find Richard, who was still out on the farm. Ten minutes later the little boy returned, in tears, on his own. He could not find his father. Eventually Richard walked in, expecting his tea. Pausing only to snatch a sandwich he and Briar's husband Sam helped Bob out to the family's Mercedes.

As Bob was carried out he asked his sister in a weak, listless voice, "Am I going to die?"

Mary, who had coped so efficiently in the previous two months, was, for once, overcome. Even now the memory of that fateful night haunts her. "I honestly thought he *was* going to die. When they had gone I staggered upstairs and was violently sick."

Bob's own views on that night show how ill he must have been. "To be honest I felt so weak I didn't care whether I lived or died."

Richard Hussey, in contrast to his brother-in-law, is a careful, considerate driver, a man who takes his time on the roads. On this occasion, however, I doubt if Stirling Moss would have driven the hundred miles or so between Wootton Bassett and Sutton faster. Much of the journey is on two motorways. "We went at speed all the way, real speed, and if we were stopped by the police then we were going to ask them to guide us in. Bob lay moaning on the front seat which was reclined as far back as it would go. He was covered with blankets and every so often he would point out a racecourse we were passing. He looked terrible with lots of spots, some of which were bleeding. He must have been very ill because it was the only time he didn't complain about my driving."

When Richard drove up to the front entrance of the hospital a stretcher was already waiting to take Bob straight to the Pinkham ward. There he was immediately put on massive antibiotics administered intravenously. His temperature was 105 degrees.

"It was quite a close thing," says Jenny. "If he'd come back two or three hours later it might have been too late."

Patients can die very quickly from septicaemia, within a matter of hours, when there is no resistance at all to infection. Blood poisoning is a real emergency and has to be treated fast. Normally if someone has an infection doctors grow the organism, prove what's causing it and then treat it. But in the case of septicaemia they don't have time to do that. They cannot wait to grow the organism that is causing the problem. Dr Jane Merrow explains: "You have to start with whatever antibiotics are known at that time to be effective. All patients who are having intensive chemotherapy have the same problem. If there aren't any white cells left in the blood then you can't fight infection."

Once the antibiotics began to work the danger to Bob's life was over. His temperature returned to normal within twenty-four hours and, though he was able to ring Mary late on Monday, he was kept in hospital for a further four days on a sustained course of antibiotics to ensure the infection did not return. His blood count was so low that on Tuesday 9th October, two days after he was rushed back to hospital, he was given a concentrated transfusion of four units of red blood cells containing the equivalent of four pints of blood. Within a few days his mouth ulcers had gone and the spots on his face and neck had dried up. Bob has no illusions about his narrow escape.

Throughout the illness the only time I really thought I was going to die was that night they took me back to hospital. I've been told since that it was touch and go whether I survived the night. Yet once the panic was over that was one spell in hospital I didn't mind. You see I wasn't on the antibiotics for very long each day so I could wander around freely without any restraint.

On Friday 12th October Bob had recovered sufficiently to be allowed home for a brief rest before the start of the fourth treatment. Monty Court picked him up in the morning and drove him to Ascot races where they were due to be met by Richard Hussey. Monty's car, in urgent need of repair, chugged along at no more than thirty miles an hour with smoke and fumes pouring into the interior. "My car was hardly the ideal conveyance for someone in Bob's condition," Monty confesses, "and I was worried we would break down and have to wait for help. But luckily we made it."

Bob's welcome home was even warmer than usual but the fright that they had all experienced had left its mark. Says Mary, "Bob was so worried he expected us to take his temperature every two minutes. If he had the slightest temperature he would persuade Richard to ring the hospital to see if they wanted him to go back in. Subconsciously we were all waiting for the signs of blood poisoning to appear again but happily it didn't happen."

On Wednesday 17th October, Richard drove Bob back to hospital to begin his fourth and, he hoped, last course of treatment, but the timing caused him to miss fulfilling an important role as best man at the marriage of Derek Thompson to Jane McLaren, daughter of the BBC's superb, knowledgeable rugby commentator Bill McLaren.

Considering Bob's performance as an usher at another close friend's wedding, Derek was quite brave to ask him to help out at his own. Bob, as we have explained, is not a man who spends too much time reading. So he didn't bother to look at the service sheets he handed out as he showed guests to their seats in the church. He discovered the mistake when the congregation began singing the first hymn. People on one side of the church were singing hymn 334. Those on the other side tried bravely to chant hymn 572. The culprit was Bob Champion, master usher, who had carelessly handed out to half the guests the wedding service of a couple married in the church earlier in the day.

Derek Thompson was horrified. "As they began to sing I heard this terrible jangling noise. I just stood there and cringed. When I got married in October 1979, I didn't dare ask Bob to be usher so he had to be best man. We all hoped he would be able to make it but on the day he was in hospital and far too ill to travel to Scotland."

Bob Champion, however, was not forgotten at the wedding. Derek proposed an emotional toast to his speedy recovery to full health and a little later a telegram arrived from the absent best man. "Sorry I can't be with you but I have to stay in hospital to look after the nurses," it read.

Bob's fourth course of treatment left him ill and demoralized but he was encouraged by the thought that it was almost certainly his last stay in hospital. He also leaned heavily on the experience of a loyal friend Julie Opperman who had suffered from cancer in the past. Bob had once rented a cottage at Marlborough owned by Mike and Julie Opperman. While he was in hospital he would often ring Julie for advice and reassurance and she more than anyone else was able to help him understand and cope with the implications of his illness. She was a great help.

Julie was the most tremendous comfort, but even she could not help at times. Those six days were as bad as ever. I was constantly sick, felt dreadful and was weaker than ever. Each cycle of treatment used to knock me down and then build me up again. After four bouts I didn't think I could go any lower. I used to lie there counting the days and telling all the hospital staff I wouldn't be coming back again whatever the doctors said. By then I'd had enough of hospital for life.

A welcome surprise was the delivery of a case of champagne from an old friend Geoffrey Greenwood, a businessman and racehorse owner. Bob had won on several horses owned by him in the past and Geoffrey hoped the bubbly might cheer him up. Geoffrey's chauffeur, a chirpy former jockey Geoff Shoemark, had ridden against Bob many times and was delighted to be asked to deliver the present to the hospital. Geoff takes up the story:

"I carried the case of champagne up to the ward, and asked to see Bob and was directed to a room at the end of the corridor. I walked past several beds but couldn't see him anywhere and was just about to leave when a voice called out weakly, 'Hello Geoff, what are you doing here?' It was Bob. I'd walked right past him without recognizing him. He looked dreadful—so ill, like a ghost. But he was pleased to see me and we had a chat about the old times. Although he was very ill it was obvious he couldn't wait to leave hospital."

John Gobourn was thoroughly intrigued at the way Bob managed to spend one night less at the hospital than other cancer patients having the same chemotherapy treatment.

"Bob and I started on the drip at exactly the same time yet he always finished several hours in front of me, just enough to leave early in the evening of day 5 while I had to wait to go home until the following morning, day 6. Eventually he told me that he had found a way of tampering with the valve on the drip so that the liquid would pass through the cannula much more quickly. He simply opened up the valve to let more liquid through and, of course, the bag then emptied much faster. It just shows how desperate he was to leave. We both dreaded the thought of any more treatment. The nurses on the ward were all fantastic and so dedicated. They knew exactly how to handle us. I think they realized Bob was fiddling with the drip but didn't say anything because they knew the thought of leaving a bit earlier cheered him up."

Bob left hospital on Monday 22nd October in a brighter frame of mind. Despite the most agonizing side effects and the crisis caused by blood poisoning he had survived four courses of treatment. Now he could plan his recovery. It was explained to him that he would have a month's rest before a re-assessment of his progress. If tests showed that the tumour had disappeared completely he would not need any more treatment. If there were still some traces then he could expect to start a course of radiation as an out-patient.

For the first few days at the farm he was still far too ill for any celebrations. He spent most of the time in bed, suffering acute stomach cramp from constipation. But early in November his condition improved so rapidly that Richard and Mary felt able to go ahead with their plans to take their two children to Miami for a fortnight's holiday. Towards the end of the first week in November Bob began driving again. He would visit friends and though he still looked dreadful he felt much better.

15th November was a momentous day. Doctors at the hospital

had always encouraged patients to continue their normal activities
as much as possible provided they felt strong enough. Now Bob
decided to ride again for the first time in months. The mount he
chose was Emma's grey pony, Henry, just 13½ hands high. It was
an emotional experience for everyone at the farm. Although riding
would clearly be a useful, beneficial therapy, Bob had also been
warned of the dangers of falling and banging his head. His blood
count was still low and there was a risk that if he cut his head in a fall
it might have been difficult to stem the flow of blood.

Hesitantly he climbed on to Henry's back, then encouraged the
pony to walk and trot through a gate into the nearest field. They
cantered twice round the field and even jumped a couple of tree
trunks. Bob rode triumphantly back to the delighted group standing
at the gate and nearly collapsed as he dismounted.

> I was knackered. My legs were like jelly and I had to go in the
> house and sit down for half an hour. I had no strength or muscles
> left and was puffing like an old man.

The next morning Bob drove the Hussey family to Heathrow
airport to catch the flight to Miami. He waved goodbye then drove
the short distance to Ascot racecourse where Kybo, the horse he
considered the best he had ever ridden, was running in the Hurst
Park Novices' Chase against another brilliant young horse, Drusus.
After Richard Rowe had gained a narrow victory on Kybo, Bob was
whisked away to be interviewed on the BBC 2 televised racing
programme by Richard Pitman. The two men, old friends, discus-
sed Kybo's performance and Bob's progress since he left hospital.
Pale, thin and cold, Bob certainly did not look a picture of health
but he left viewers in no doubt about his determination to be back in
time for the Grand National.

On 19th November, he enjoyed a rare night out in London at the
finals of the Stable Lads' Boxing tournament, an annual function at
the World Sporting Club which raises a considerable amount of
money for the Stable Lads' Welfare Trust. The wine and brandy,
alas, proved a little too much for Bob's system the following morning: when he returned to hospital for a series of exhaustive tests, the
alcohol level in his blood was too high to take an accurate reading.

He returned for a second test the following day and also had a body scan and lung function tests.

While the Hussey family was away Bob was on his own for the first time in months. Typically his first move was to import a girlfriend to look after him, and he also spent some time staying with friends. Already he was feeling stronger. Still determined to be fit to ride Aldaniti in the Grand National he decided to start riding racehorses again at exercise. For three mornings running he returned to his old routine of riding out for Paul Cole, the brightest young trainer in Lambourn. Cole, who trains flat racehorses, was anxious that Bob should not do too much too soon and confined him to walking and trotting horses on the roads. On the second morning the two riders nearest to Bob both fell heavily on the road. Tommy Jennings, an experienced former jockey, escaped with a few bruises but the other rider, a middle-aged amateur, was not so lucky. He suffered a badly broken thigh and other injuries. Bob found the effort of riding out in the mornings far more tiring than he had anticipated and so, after three days, sensibly decided to wait until he was much stronger:

> The sight of those two crashing down on the road made me realize I might be the next one. They were both much fitter than me.

Before the end of the month there was time to stay with his new regular girlfriend Jenny and her parents, and to visit other friends. The moment of re-assessment and decision was near and though Bob felt much better, the crucial meeting with his doctors on 29th November was constantly on his mind.

> To be honest, I was frightened. I'd had so many injections and so much treatment in the last few months that I couldn't face the thought of any more.

Chapter 9

BOB STAYED WITH Derek Thompson at Walton-on-Thames at the end of the month and the pair drove together to hospital for Bob's appointment with Dr Jane Merrow on 29th November. At first she seemed encouraging. Bob's progress in four courses of treatment had been excellent, she said. Tests showed that the tumour in his chest had gone but there was a possibility that the fibrous tissue around it might still contain a few lingering malignant cells. The choice for Bob was an agonizing one. He could start a course of radiation treatment, which would almost certainly damage his lungs further; or he could have two more courses of chemotherapy treatment.

Dr Merrow explained the dilemma we faced. She understood my feelings and was always very open with me. If I had not wanted to ride again she would have been happy for me to have the radiation. But she explained that the combination of drugs followed by radiation produces more lung damage than drugs alone. Even more than the usual 33 per cent.

"If he did go ahead with radiation at that point then he would certainly not have been able to go back to race riding," Dr Merrow confirmed. He had done well on the drugs and so it seemed reasonable to continue with them and give him two more treatments to consolidate the tremendous progress he had already made.

The inevitable decision, then, that Bob should have two more courses of chemotherapy was a joint one between the patient and his doctor but it left Bob in a critically low state of depression. He had convinced himself he would not need any further treatment and the news that he had to go through so much more was like a prison sentence.

It was a terrible blow. I was heartbroken. If I'd been anyone else I'd have been able to have radiation as an outpatient. It just made me even more determined to ride again and if that meant two more treatments then I was prepared to go through with it. Even so I was bitter with everyone and everything; for the first and only time in my life I started hitting the bottle in a desperate attempt to forget. Brandy, wine, anything—you name it. Over the next few days, at least, I think it worked. Most of the time I had too much drink inside me to care. But once I was back in hospital I couldn't face tea, let alone alcohol.

The very next day, 30th November, fate dealt Bob Champion another vicious stroke. Distressed and unhappy, nursing a king-sized hangover after an uncharacteristic night of drinking, he turned up at Sandown racecourse to see Aldaniti run for the first time during the season and watched in disbelief as the horse was pulled up near the finish hopping lame. As Richard Rowe led him back to a disconsolate group under the trees by the racecourse stables it was clear he had broken down badly again on the same foreleg as before.

Josh Gifford was sure the horse was gone for good. "This time it was so severe that I was convinced he would not run again," he says. And even if Aldaniti did recover he would be out of action for at least a year. Bob's passport to a famous comeback in the 1980 Grand National had been withdrawn in the cruellest of circumstances. But one more disappointment was not going to succeed where so much suffering and pain had failed. Biting back his own feelings of despair Bob somehow forced a smile and told Valda Embiricos, "Never mind, we'll just have to come back together."

The meanest bookmaker in the business would readily have offered long odds about that particular forecast coming true. Aldaniti's tendon was so seriously damaged that it was put in a plaster cast for three weeks before an operation to pin-fire the injury was carried out by the vet Mike Ashton. The horse returned to Barkfold Manor Stud once more for a prolonged rest, but this time even the vet was extremely pessimistic about his prospects of running again.

By the end of that calamitous day's racing at Sandown, Bob's mood was suicidal.

> I don't think I could have taken any more. When you are a jump jockey you are used to things going terribly wrong but this was too much. Looking back at it now I don't think I was sane at the time. I behaved very strangely.

Derek Thompson once more provided refuge for his friend that night and the next morning Bob collected the Hussey family at Heathrow. The date, 1st December, was two days after Emma's eighth birthday but no-one in the family felt much like celebrating. Somehow the dismal weekend passed and on Monday 3rd December Richard drove Bob back to hospital at Sutton to begin his fifth course of chemotherapy treatment. It proved to be the worst of all.

> I didn't think it was possible to feel any worse, but this time I had never been so ill in my life. Perhaps it was the effect of the drugs on me after a rest. Mentally I was in a terrible state. Aldaniti's lameness made me give up fighting for a couple of weeks.
>
> The Grand National had been a goal, a target for me to aim at. Once Aldaniti was out I knew I wouldn't ride again that season and so gave up all hope. That was the hardest time, the closest I came to giving up.
>
> I'd lie in bed heaving and retching for hour after hour with virtually nothing coming up. In the end it became so painful on my chest and throat that I'd sip a bit of tea or Coke so that at least something would come out. I was in a ward surrounded by others who were just as ill. We hardly spoke at all. If you are as sick as that every day you don't feel like being very friendly. You are so down you don't take any notice of other people.
>
> The sweat poured off me and set off another chain reaction because the smell of your own body and that horrible liquid platinum makes you vomit again.

Frank Pullen, that most loyal of friends, kept up his daily vigil but for the first time became seriously worried at Bob's state of mind. "I remember that week I rang Josh Gifford up one day and said 'You must go and see Bob, I don't think he'll last through the weekend.' Bob lay there groaning and kept pleading, 'Please let me die, Frank. Tell them to leave me alone.' I gave him a right mouthful. I told him, 'Do you think I've come all this way to hear you talk like that?' I told him he couldn't let down his family and friends after such a long fight.''

Frank would sit patiently by Bob's bedside, wipe his mouth and face when he was sick, and now and then empty the bowl.

Another anxious visitor that week was Monty Court. Usually Bob showed some signs of welcome but this time he lay morosely, his back turned. Monty passed him the evening paper. With a great effort Bob turned to the racing results then groaned, "I've missed another bloody winner."

Monty Court, a fine joke teller, now produced two of his very best in a determined effort to lift Bob's mood. Both fell on stony ground without a flicker of interest from the patient. Desperate now, Monty told Bob how his car nearly had not started and that he might not have been able to visit that evening.

Says Monty: "Bob was lying on his right side near the window and from there you could look out and see some trees without any leaves. It was a dark, miserable night, with no lights on in his room. The only light in the ward was that coming from the corridor. He didn't say anything at all, just lay there, a forlorn, heaving, miserable dejected figure."

Finally Bob muttered feebly, "Hey, Monty."

"Yes, Bob."

"Would you do me a favour?"

"Yes, of course, anything you ask," answered Monty, eager to please him in any way possible.

"Please leave me alone."

Monty is far too experienced a Fleet Street journalist to take offence at such an unlikely request. He muttered his farewells then left the ward.

"I think only those of us who saw Bob in hospital realize just how ill he was," he recalls. "That particular time was the worst. Imagine how he must have felt. All the time in hospital he put up the most tremendous fight but on this occasion things were just too much for him. He's never been the greatest conversationalist and that day talking to him was as bad as pulling teeth.

"After that visit I was sure he wouldn't ride again. To be absolutely honest I thought if he wanted to ride again it would be a very brave man who allowed him to have a licence. We all have an ignorance of cancer but the risks and hazards of his particular sport are hardly an ideal form of recuperation from such a critical illness."

Carol, too, had her doubts about Bob riding again: "When he returned for his fifth course his lung function tests were very important. Obviously his lungs had already been affected by the drugs but we didn't know to what extent they had been permanently damaged. We had never had anyone who needed the maximum use of their lungs again."

The constant injection of drugs into his body finally proved too much. All week Bob had been extending his hour break early in the morning by five and then ten minutes. "He would have gone nuts if he didn't have that little break," says Jenny.

On Thursday morning he summoned Carol and told her bluntly that he wanted to be taken off the drip, permanently. He made it clear he did not wish to continue with the treatment. The demand was not a surprise to Carol, an experienced ward sister. Many patients, demoralized and weakened by the endless treatment, have reached the same point of despair. In America, where some patients are treated continuously with chemotherapy for as much as two years, doctors prescribe heroin in small amounts to lift their spirits when they have become so run down mentally and physically that they cannot take any more.

"There's no point in arguing with a patient who feels like Bob," Carol says. "The best way to handle the problem is to send them off for a walk round the hospital and advise them to consider the consequences of their action. If you argue and try to persuade them to change their minds you merely make them more determined to give up. They usually come back after an hour when they've had time to think things through, and ask to be re-connected. Some feel they need a week off but they all come back in the end. They realize they have no choice if they want to live."

Free at last of the drip and its constant attendant, the stanchion,

Bob wandered off on his own round the hospital. The sense of freedom at once bucked his spirits. Eventually he found himself in the children's ward and talked to several young patients, some only three or four years old, but all of them bald from the effects of the chemotherapy treatment. Some were suffering from cancer, others from leukaemia. All seemed remarkably cheerful. Bob left the room with tears in his eyes and returned to the Pinkham ward.

> It was a very important lesson in my life. There was I moaning and groaning at the nurses and everyone, thinking only of myself, and downstairs those poor little kids were going through the same thing without complaining. Seeing them was the turning point for me. If they could take the treatment then so could I.

"He came back looking very thoughtful and a little bit embarrassed," Carol recalls, "and asked me very quietly to put the drip back on. All the patients feel the same as him at some point and at least fifty per cent do come off the drip for a while."

Bob left hospital early on the evening of Saturday 8th December at the end of the fifth course and though he was desperately ill there was a perceptible lift in his mood as we drove westwards down the M4 that night. He even persuaded me to stop at a call-box and ring his sister Mary so that she would have three hamburgers waiting as we reached the farmhouse. However ill he felt during the week he was able able to eat one good meal on his release before the onset of crippling constipation. As we sped away from the hospital he said:

> The worst should be over. I'm counting the days to the end of the treatment. They've done their best to kill me but they won't succeed now. I'm almost there.

Even so he retired to bed for the next three days and when he returned to hospital on day 9, Wednesday, 12th December, his doctors were sufficiently worried about a slight cold that they insisted he should stay under their care until the weekend.

> That was the best time of all in hospital. The doctors were anxious that I might have blood poisoning again and just wanted to keep

an eye on me. I had two days there without any drips, injections or treatment apart from some rough old cough mixture. I was free to wander where I liked, watch television, pester my friends with phone calls and chat to the nurses.

The Pinkham ward was full at the time so I slept each night in the Kennaway ward, a floor below. It was the ward I'd waited in for hours at the start of my illness. Now I didn't mind staying there at all. It was still full of very old, very sick patients and that just made me thankful that I was so much younger and had nearly finished my courses of treatment.

Bob returned home at the weekend in the middle of a crisis. Four horses had escaped from a field and had galloped onto the main road. One of them—Henry, Emma's pony—had been hit and killed by a car. The other three were caught safely but Emma was distraught and Bob found their usual roles reversed as he, for once, was able to comfort her.

He visited hospital once more for injections on day 16 when the decision was taken that he would be able to spend Christmas with his family then start his sixth course of treatment on Boxing Day.

There was a moment of rare humour in December when a northern trainer John Bingham, unaware of Bob's illness and his prolonged absence from the racecourse, rang to offer him a ride on one of his runners at Southwell later in the week. "That bucked me up," smiles Bob. "I'd never ridden for him before and it was nice to know I was still wanted."

Towards the end of the cycle, Bob, as usual, began to feel much better and Christmas at the farm was much more cheerful than anyone could have anticipated in the previous months. Bob's parents came to stay and he was inundated with presents, cards and telegrams. Best of all was a gift of a thousand pounds from Josh Gifford and his owners. When Josh had first learned of Bob's grave illness he had promised to give him his usual retainer. It was a characteristically generous gesture by the trainer. He wrote to all his owners, collected over seven hundred pounds from them and topped the figure up to a thousand pounds himself. "It was the very least I could do in the circumstances," Josh says.

Bob also received a large get well card from Aldaniti. It was sent to him by Alexandra Embiricos, daughter of the horse's owners, and many of her friends at school. Alexandra organized an Aldaniti Fan Club at her school, charged a minimal subscription fee and sent the proceeds to Bob each Christmas for the Injured Jockeys Fund.

Bob set off for hospital on 26th December in a surprisingly bright mood. His final course of chemotherapy treatment was by far the easiest thanks to the devotion and persistence of his favourite nurse, Jenny. Disappointed that the usual tranquillizing drugs had not worked on him Jenny determined to discover another method to help him sleep. Says Bob:

> The first thing she tried on that sixth course was a drug that puts the children out. She told me I'd go out at once too but, as usual, I didn't. I seemed to be immune.

Doggedly Jenny tried yet another concoction and, to her delight and relief, it worked. Within minutes Bob was asleep.

> This time I was knocked right out; for the first time I slept so well that I was hardly ever awake to be sick. I was drowsy all the time which is the best way to be. I was counting the days by then and that helped to make the whole thing easier.

Towards the end of the treatment there was a scare when swellings suddenly appeared on both of Bob's nipples, and for a few hours he was in a state of panic. A doctor examined him and decided that tests should be taken at once to decide the cause of the swelling.

> It put the fear of God up me. One of the doctors thought it might indicate the treatment had not worked properly, but after they examined my blood they decided it was just another side effect of the treatment. Apparently it occurs quite frequently. The swellings, curiously, lasted until the summer.

Bob left the Royal Marsden Hospital at Sutton for the last time on New Year's Day, 1980. The date seemed a good omen. As we drove down the motorway he was adamant he would not return for more treatment, whatever the tests showed.

I'm not going back and that's it. I've had as much as I can take. If they can't cure me with the huge amount of drugs they've already put through me then they are unlikely to succeed by giving me even more. I'll never have chemotherapy again, never.

Chapter 10

THE FIRST WEEK after Bob's final course of chemotherapy treatment was impossibly difficult to bear. He lay in bed, seriously ill, wondering at times if he would ever recover. He was frequently sick and suffered the usual torturous constipation: in addition painful sores appeared in his mouth and face and he sweated profusely. His weight dropped to just below nine stone.

> I was so weak I could barely stand up long enough to reach the bathroom. My muscles had all wasted away and I looked like an old man. Each treatment seemed to knock me down a bit lower and by the end of the last one I was so feeble I didn't care about anything. I'd just about given up.

Dottie Channing-Williams called to see Bob before she left with her family for a holiday in Barbados. The visit was a mistake as far as she was concerned because she spent the entire holiday wondering if Bob would still be alive when she returned to England. "I can't describe just how ill he looked and I doubted if he would live very much longer. That was the worst I saw him through the illness. I took my daughter Nicole with me but was so shocked by the way he looked that I wouldn't let her see him. At that point he didn't care tuppence for himself. He just lay there groaning. He didn't talk, he didn't even move. The smell was awful. I rang Mary two or three times while we were away and when I came back Bob was a different person."

The crisis had passed. On day 9, 5th January, Bob was too ill to travel back to hospital for the usual injections and tests as part of his sixth course of treatment. Richard Hussey felt he had improved enough over the weekend to justify a trip to the hospital on 7th

January; Bob was able to have an injection of bleomycin that day but was still too unwell to take any tests. So he returned to the hospital yet again on 9th January.

> I was bad. All that treatment had just about finished me. I was drained of all my strength and energy. There was nothing left. If they had forced me to have any more chemotherapy I can't imagine that I would have survived. I was as low as you can possibly go and it took me far longer than I had expected to recover. During the first half of January I was just like a new-born baby who had to be washed and cleaned several times a day. I didn't have the energy to do anything for myself and all the time I was dreading the assessment the doctors had to make at the end of the month.

Towards the end of January Bob began to feel a little better. He would walk round the farmhouse for five or ten minutes each day and send the odd telex message for Richard but he was still so tired that he was asleep in bed soon after seven each evening.

Richard and Mary were both acutely aware how close Bob had been to dying. Now they tried to persuade him to pace his recovery steadily and to consider other options if he was unable to ride again. Several close friends, too, urged him to contemplate a new career. Riding over fences, they argued, was quite simply too dangerous for someone who had just recovered from cancer. Those of us who had marvelled at his tremendous, prolonged fight against cancer and the appalling effects of the treatment to cure it were anxious that he should not risk returning to hospital with injuries from a race fall caused by resuming riding too quickly. Bob treated such well intentioned suggestions with scorn. Aware that regaining his jockey's licence might be a problem, he sought and gained the immediate support of Peter Smith, the backbone for so many years of the Jockeys' Association.

> Peter told me that once I was fully fit the Jockeys' Association would fight for my right to ride again with all the power at their disposal. Mind you, the way I felt at the time I couldn't imagine being fully fit for another six months.

"I've never known anyone as determined as Bob," Richard Hussey says. "He was going to ride again whatever the consequences and nothing anyone could say would make him consider other alternatives. If it had been me I would have said to hell with riding. But Bob was so single minded; the sheer strength of his determination was frightening because there were times when we wondered if he would be given a licence again. I dread to think of the fuss he would have made if they had tried to stop him. One night when he was very ill he repeated that he would rather be killed in a race fall than die a lingering death in hospital. And he meant it. He became quite dramatic about it."

Mary laughed. "As soon as he was a little better he'd go outside and jog to the cottages a hundred yards or so away. It was the funniest sight—this bald-headed fool in his dressing-gown and slippers tottering along the farm track chased by a barking dog. We all laughed at him. Of course we did! Once he'd finished his treatment and he was cleared he changed his tune and it was not quite so important to him to come back in such a hurry. He realized he was going to need to be a hundred and ten per cent fit before he ever tried to ride in a race again."

On 18th January, suitably encouraged by his faltering attempts at jogging, Bob returned to Hungerford Squash Club for his first session of treatment with Val Ridgeway, the club's skilled remedial masseuse. Val had been used to patching up Bob from the effects of falls in previous years but was now shaken by his emaciated, hollow cheeked appearance:

"I knew he had been ill with cancer and feared the worst until he sent me a message from hospital saying he planned to start exercises again sometime in January. When he came to me he was in a hell of a state, and quite unable to do anything at all. His muscles had completely wasted away. They were pathetic little things. Any normal seven-year-old would have been stronger and he was too weak to do his own exercises.

"I worked on the muscles with body massage and at first he was far too feeble to do anything strenuous. His back was in a terrible state and his arms were useless. He was just skin and bone. The muscles were just about still there but so tight. They all had to be loosened up. Yet from the start even when he was lying there in a useless state he was insistent that he would ride again. The only thing in his favour was that he had always been a fighter. In the past I had seen him ride in a terrible condition after some punishing falls. He didn't like giving in to pain."

On 20th January Bob left the Husseys to stay for a few days with his girlfriend Jenny. On the twenty-fourth he returned to hospital for yet more tests, including a body scan, and stayed the night with his parents at Lingfield. The next morning he was given a comprehensive lung function examination to determine just how seriously his breathing had been affected by the drug bleomycin.

Various wires were taped to his heart and lungs as he breathed and puffed into different instruments before a tiring session on a treadmill. He finished the tests totally exhausted. Later in the day he returned to the Husseys' farm and after a family debate made the crucial decision to move back to his own house the very next day.

It was not an easy choice. Richard and Mary were anxious that he should stay with them for another week or two until he was stronger. But Bob's house had been empty for almost six months; he was worried about the problems of damp and the mystery of diesel oil disappearing from the tank. He felt well enough to assert his independence and, significantly, resolved to move a few days before he would learn the doctors' vital assessment on the progress of his treatment.

So Bob moved back home on 26th January.

No-one else could have looked after me like Richard, Mary and the children. They were all terrific. Mary knew how to handle me. When I felt sorry for myself she would bully me. But once my health started to improve I realized if I was going to resume riding then it was time I learned to stand on my own two feet again. Staying with Richard and Mary any longer would have been the easy way out.

Bob's return home quickly reduced most of the village's telephone system to a shambles. In previous years he had used an Ansafone machine to record messages while he was away. Now, far too impatient to wait for the installation engineer and anxious not to miss any calls, Bob, with the aid of a complicated instruction book, wired up the Ansafone then set off on a shopping expedition to collect some essential supplies. When he arrived back he discovered that the hour-long tape on the Ansafone had been completely used. How pleasant, he reflected, that so many of his friends had taken the trouble to ring during his absence.

Imagine his surprise and annoyance when he wound back the tape and listened to a series of garbled messages and conversations between people he didn't know. Somehow his Ansafone had picked up and faithfully recorded the telephone calls of most of the numbers in the village. There was not a single communication for him on the tape.

Bob spent the next few days worrying about his appointment with his doctors on 31st January. The fear of bad news kept him awake in the final few nights. He would drift into a disturbed, restless sleep then suffer nightmares that he was back in hospital on the drip. He need not have worried. The latest tests showed that the malignant tumour in his chest had gone, and the final two treatments had cleared up any remaining malignant particles in the fibrous tissues around the mass. He would not need radiation. His nightmare was over. There was just one minor concern. The doctors warned him that his lung function tests showed that his breathing had been impaired by the bleomycin. The full extent of the damage was not clear but it might be a problem when he was fit enough to resume riding. Dr Jane Merrow points out, "A lot of our patients are so thankful to have made it that nothing else in life seems important. Bob was different. He was always certain he would race again and the news that his lungs were damaged made him more determined than ever to prove us wrong."

Although still very weak Bob ran from the hospital to his car in a mood of wild elation. Now he was ready to start his fight to regain fitness. He stopped at a telephone box to ring his mother and a few friends with the good news then drove home reflecting on what might have been. Ten years previously chemotherapy treatment for his particular type of cancer was not available. He was aware that if he had been ill ten years ago he would have died. Now, thanks to inventive, much improved techniques, he was cured though he knew that some patients could lapse in the first two years after the treatments. That was not a possibility he wished to consider.

Bob drove at once from London to Hungerford for a second appointment at the Squash Club with Val Ridgeway. "As you can imagine he was very pleased with himself," she recalls. "But his body didn't match his spirit and though he urgently needed regular exercise he was not ready for it. From the moment he first came to me he wanted to know exactly what percentage I thought his muscles had improved after each session. He was always aiming at being two hundred per cent fit, nothing less, and was quite fanatical about it. He had the most incredible will to succeed."

Bob visited Val twice more early in February and started going racing again. Bitterly cold, windswept racecourses at that time of year did not seem the ideal places for convalescence for such a pale, thin patient but the enjoyment of racing visibly lifted his morale. There was also time to plan a holiday in Miami in mid-February with a close friend, Ian Watkinson, whose own riding career had been ended by severe head injuries sustained in a race fall.

"We had promised ourselves a holiday when we had both recovered," says Ian, "and now Bob was fit to travel. But we made the mistake of our lives in choosing a holiday in Miami at that time of year. The whole thing was a disaster. The flight out there was too long for Bob, who was showing signs of strain in the final hours, so we stayed at a hotel close to Miami airport the first night."

In the morning the likely lads caught a taxi to Miami beach in search of possible female talent and a suitable hotel on the sea front. They failed on both counts. All the hotels in Miami were fully booked up with old age pensioners. Bob's recollections of the Florida fiasco are pretty dismal.

The average age of the people in Miami must have been ninety. There wasn't a young girl in the place. It was as if we were in a space-age film and all the young people had been swept off the planet. Miami is an ideal place if you are retired or on honeymoon and don't want any distractions.

Eventually they found a spare room in a seedy hotel far from the beach. They spent the days gloomily walking along the beach and the evenings watching television in their hotel room. When Bob left his wig off he was aware of curious and almost hostile glances in his direction. One woman asked if he belonged to the Indian religious sect that chant songs as they collect money in the street. Bob and Ian decided to hire a car but found that every available vehicle in Miami had already been booked. Bored and dispirited after four uneventful days in Miami, they agreed to return to England and took a taxi to the airport. Urged on by his two passengers—who are both immensely fast behind the wheel of a car—the hapless taxi driver began to speed past the meandering traffic in a bid to catch an earlier flight. For Bob, that brief car journey was the high spot of the holiday.

We were really flying along when we heard the sound of a police siren in pursuit. The next minute a woman cop came flashing past, forced us into the side of the road and jumped out waving a large revolver around. She looked at our driver's documents, gave us the once over and booked him. We were tickled pink.

Back in England in late February Bob started riding out again for the Lambourn trainer, Paul Cole. At first he restricted himself to walking and trotting horses on the roads but within a few days he felt strong enough to try cantering quietly. His friend Tommy Jennings viewed his initial attempts with dismay.

"Bob looked bloody awful when he started riding out again. It made me feel ill seeing him struggle on a horse. He was far too weak to be riding a quiet pony, let alone a full-blooded racehorse. Anyone else would have packed up after such a terrible ordeal in hospital but he had remarkable will power.

"He looked so bad that we were all certain it was just a question of time before he was back in hospital. Normally he had a backside on him like a double-decker bus but then he was just a skeleton and, it seemed, on borrowed time. He was unrecognizable but so persistent. He kept coming back every morning. It was bitterly cold but he had tremendous spirit."

After riding out Bob would often visit Val for much-needed massage on his aching muscles.

I was still hopelessly unfit. Even walking around at race meetings left me in pain in the evenings. Riding was all right when the horses were walking and trotting but I found cantering very difficult at first. My hands suffered badly from numbness and pins and needles, so it was awkward to hold a hard puller. My feet, too, ached and when I was tired my balance was affected.

I had very little feeling in my feet. That was another side effect of the treatment. But the worst pain of all was in my back. I'd lie in bed crying out loud with the sheer agony. The more I did in the day the worse my back became at night. But by then I was committed. I pressed on with riding and exercise each day. That was the only chance I had of regaining complete fitness.

Pete Fisher, another good friend at the Squash Club, advised Bob to take up running. Pete had already won his own prolonged battle to establish himself as an all-round athlete. So small at birth that he was not expected to live, he remained in an oxygen tent for nine months and was fed intravenously through his ankles. When he was older doctors feared he would not be strong enough to play sport. A family friend, Larry Williams, a former player for the Manchester United football team, encouraged Pete to start daily training; he became a fitness fanatic and such a good footballer that he played several hundred times for Hungerford.

Says Pete, "Larry Williams died of cancer and it was a terrible shock when I heard Bob was in hospital with the same illness. Imagine how I felt when he finished his treatment and asked me to help him regain his strength. Early on he was so weak he couldn't feel his feet or hands properly. I must say I didn't think he had recovered from the illness. He looked awful.

"That first day we went for a run of about two miles and I made him promise to stop if he felt ill. Well, he stopped three times. He looked shattered but had tremendous will power and wouldn't quit. You could see the determination on his face. It was obvious how much he wanted to finish the run but at that stage his legs weren't strong enough.

"The second run a few days later was a little easier for him and we had several more. Some of the time he would even run on the roads barefoot to try to get some feeling back in his feet. He's the most determined person I've ever met. He was always set on race riding again and he wouldn't accept anything else."

Val gave Bob a skipping rope to use at home but when he tried it in the garden he kept falling over as his legs tangled in the rope. After ten minutes he gave up the unequal struggle and consigned the skipping rope to the depths of a cupboard in the kitchen.

To be honest I'd never been able to skip properly but I didn't like to admit it to Val. So I told her I used the rope every day.

Bob returned to hospital on 28th February 1980 for the latest in a series of monthly checks. His blood tests, to his intense relief, were perfect. Early in March he drove down to Findon to stay with Josh and Althea Gifford and rode out the following morning. Althea was in the kitchen when her daughter Tina rushed into the room shouting in alarm, "Mummy, mummy, Bob's upstairs looking like a little baby." Tina had watched in awe as he'd taken off his wig and put on his crash helmet.

Josh Gifford was elated at the progress of his stable jockey: "Although Bob was still terribly weak and light he was eating well and taking a great interest in the horses. Once he was cleared by the hospital I knew he would come back because he was always so determined. He obviously had the will power to ride again so I was prepared to rely on his judgement when he thought he was ready. If he was not fit enough then I hoped and believed he would have said so. At that stage neither of us felt he should try to race ride again until the next season which started right at the end of July."

Josh Gifford, typically, plays down his part in Bob Champion's comeback from such a grave illness. Yet while his jockey languished in hospital Josh faced problems of a different nature as he kept his promise that he would not retain an outside rider. Instead he relied on his two promising young stable lads, Christy Kinane and Richard Rowe. At first both shared the rides from the stable but soon it became clear that Rowe, tough and ambitious, was a most talented jockey. Inevitably in the course of swift transition from inexperienced, unknown apprentice to successful jockey he made mistakes. One or two horses that might have won were beaten. Racegoers and the horses' owners, understandably, criticized Rowe on those occasions and there was pressure on Josh Gifford to employ a more experienced jockey. Firmly he resisted such suggestions.

"Of course there were times when I could have shouted at Richard. But you have to believe in people and I think he's the best young jockey in the country; he has the physique, the talent, the temperament. I remember only too well when I was riding the trainers who would niggle, niggle, niggle at you all the time. Well, I can be very critical but I don't hold it against my jockeys. I want my boys to go out there and put the horse, not the orders, first.

"I was prepared to back my faith in Richard. We all make mistakes in life and he did very well when you consider how he was rushed into the job. I had given my word to Bob and I had no intention of going back on it. Luckily we had a really good season with a steady supply of winners. Things would have been much more difficult for me if we'd had a bad run."

In the second week of March Bob enjoyed a brief new role as a commentator for BBC radio. Derek Thompson's suggestion that the BBC should use Bob's expertise at the major National Hunt festival at Cheltenham was readily approved by his Sports Editor. During the three days at Cheltenham Bob was interviewed several times by Peter Bromley and Ray Moore. Derek was pleasantly surprised by the way Bob took his new job. "He was really very good— surprisingly good when you consider he is usually a bit shy and self-conscious. He spoke with authority and good sense about the leading horses and jockeys and gave the programme an interesting and different point of view."

Bob's resolution to ride again was given a significant and generous boost by an old friend, Anthony Robinson, who owned several good horses and rode some of them in races with much enthusiasm and dash. Anthony told Bob that he had been so seriously ill with cancer three years earlier that he had required major surgery. Even so he had been determined to resume riding as an amateur jockey and he actively encouraged Bob to continue with his plans to resume his former career.

Anthony Robinson's comeback after a most difficult and major operation to win the 1979 Irish Distillers Grand National on his own horse Tied Cottage was a feat of quite oustanding bravery and endurance. It was not generally known that the effects of that operation were sufficient for the English authorities to decline to renew his amateur's licence. Undaunted, and showing his usual vigour and enterprise, Anthony merely changed his tactics, applied for an Irish riding licence and received it in time to partner Tied Cottage at Fairyhouse in April 1979 in the Irish Grand National.

In his previous race Tied Cottage had fallen at the last fence in the 1979 Tote Cheltenham Gold Cup while disputing the lead with the winner, Alverton. At Fairyhouse, certainly, the horse was much fitter than the jockey. Together Tied Cottage and his intrepid owner led at a roaring gallop for more than three miles until headed at the second last fence by Tommy Carmody on Prince Rock. It seemed the brilliant young professional's strength and expertise would prove decisive in a tight finish. Prince Rock held a slender lead at the final fence but was immediately challenged again on the run-in by Tied Cottage and his tired but gallant owner. Stylish is certainly not the first adjective that leaps to mind about Anthony Robinson's riding, but years of experience had made him pretty effective in a finish. Close to exhaustion, he called for a final supreme effort from Tied Cottage and gained the response he so fully deserved. Tied Cottage battled on like a hero and together they gained a famous victory by a neck from Prince Rock. Typically Anthony avoided any publicity and insisted that his illness should not be mentioned.

At Cheltenham a year later in March 1980, Anthony showed Bob a letter from his own specialist confirming that he was fit to ride and promised full support if Bob found any difficulty in obtaining his licence from the Jockey Club. No man could have been more pleased, then, than Bob Champion on the Thursday of the Cheltenham meeting when he was able to describe on the radio the superb win of his friend's horse Tied Cottage, ridden by Tommy Carberry, in the most important steeplechase of the year, the Tote Cheltenham Gold Cup. Extremely unlucky in the 1979 race and second in 1977, Tied Cottage, at the advanced age of twelve, finally gained his reward for persistence with a marvellous all-the-way victory to the immense delight of his owner and his many friends. How cruel that a marginal amount of contaminated feed in his system should have led to his subsequent disqualification many weeks later on technical grounds.

Typically Anthony Robinson took that stunning reverse with
philosophical calm. Showing an admirable blend of magnanimity
and good humour he turned up at Warwick racecourse in June to
help present the coveted Gold Cup, which had been his for such a
short while, to Arthur Barrow, the owner of Master Smudge, the
runner-up to Tied Cottage at Cheltenham. Afterwards the two men
shared a bottle of champagne in the bar. Bob admired Anthony
Robinson enormously.

He was a terrific support. He had kept the knowledge of his illness
a close secret but he made a point of telling me all about it, and his
comeback from a similar kind of illness gave me fresh heart. He
could not have been more helpful. I was thrilled when his horse
won the Gold Cup and couldn't believe it when I heard the news
that he was eventually disqualified.

The week after the Cheltenham meeting Bob stayed with Ian
Watkinson at Newmarket and rode out on several mornings for two
trainers, Tom Jones and David Morley. It was not a happy experience. The very first morning the horse he rode came unpleasantly
close to carting him right across the famous Heath.

The trouble was that I just didn't have any strength in my arms,
legs or tummy. This particular horse was not considered a hard or
dangerous ride, but I had a hell of a job holding him and when we
pulled up I was puffing like an express train. My wind was not at
all good and I was beginning to wonder if I'd ever regain full
fitness. The cold, damp weather didn't help so I decided it might
be wiser to go to the warmer climate of America for the spring
and summer. Josh seemed to think it was a good idea so I
arranged to fly over at the beginning of April.

First he had two important dates in England in the last week of
March. On Thursday 27th March he travelled once more to hospital
for his regular monthly tests—which proved satisfactory—and then
he dashed up to Liverpool where the BBC were employing him
again for the Grand National meeting. The high spot of the three
days was an interview he recorded with Derek Thompson as they

walked round the course examining the daunting fences. Bob explained the hazards, pitfalls and excitement of riding round Aintree and the twelve-minute interview proved to be the cornerstone of the BBC's radio racing programme on Saturday. In addition Bob was interviewed by Judith Chalmers and gave several on-the-spot assessments during other races.

While he was at Liverpool Bob sat fully clothed on the weighing-room scales and was astonished to find his weight had soared to 12 stone 9 pounds.

I'd never been as heavy as that in my life! It was a good sign that I was recovering. I knew my weight had increased because my clothes were becoming tight but 12 stone 9 pounds—that meant I'd put on almost four stone in the three months since I left hospital! I made bloody sure it didn't go any higher. Obviously I missed riding at Liverpool, but if I was not ready to take part then the next best thing was to be paid by the BBC to be there. I had every intention of riding in the 1981 Grand National. On Aldaniti, of course.

Chapter 11

ONE VITAL CONFIDENCE-boosting set of equipment was missing from Bob's baggage when he flew to America on 1st April. Encouraged by the growth of a few, soft, wispy hairs on his head he had abandoned his impressive collection of wigs. It was a decision he bitterly regretted as the massive Jumbo jet clawed its way into the sky above Heathrow.

By leaving the wigs behind I knew I would have to face people without any camouflage. But as we sat on the runway some of the passengers gave me some funny looks and I thought, Christ, I've made a mistake. I should have brought a wig with me. I was terribly self-conscious about being bald. More than you can imagine. But I reasoned it might not be quite so bad in America because I didn't know that many people there.

My theory was that my hair would grow quicker in the fresh air than hidden under a wig. Basically I was going to the States to ride and it's too uncomfortable to wear a wig under a crash helmet. It's too hot and doesn't fit properly.

Bob flew from Heathrow to New York and then caught another plane to Camden, South Carolina, where Burly Cocks's horses spend the winter months. The temperature in Camden was noticeably warmer. Bob stayed three weeks at the training centre as a work jockey, riding several horses each morning before embarking on a daily series of strenuous muscle-building exercises at a superbly equipped health spa in Camden.

Burly Cocks, a delightful old character who has been training racehorses since 1940, was pleased to welcome back his English protégé. "Ah, that Bob," he says in rasping, gravelly tones, "is a

116

regular guy. A very presentable fellow, tremendously popular here, full of fun, very obliging and good company. The girls chase him all over the place. He has a quiet way with him. Bob had been in touch with me and explained he thought our warmer climate would help him recover more quickly and we were thrilled to see him again though he sure looked ill when he arrived early in April.

"At first he couldn't do much on a horse. He used to get tired very quickly. But he didn't miss a day's work. He was a bit self-conscious when he arrived without his wig but he didn't look too much out of place. A lot of fellows out here don't have any hair either."

The routine at Camden was a punishing one. Bob would ride three or four horses each morning on the circular sand training track before moving on to the health spa. There he would tackle a series of exercising machines, bicycles, running machines, chest expanders and gadgets to tone up the muscles in his arms, legs, stomach and back. Then followed ten minutes in the sauna and fifteen minutes in a whirlpool. Then more work on weights and mechanical pulleys. Most days he would go running too. Bob will always be grateful to the trainer Burly Cocks.

From the start Burly put me on the very best horses in his stables—some of the best jumpers in America. Zaccio, who won the Eclipse Award for the best steeplechaser, was the first horse I sat on when I arrived at Camden. The next was Winter Wonderland, who won four races on the bounce. I appreciated Burly's faith in me. That gave me more heart than anything.

Even so it took such a long time for my wind to come right. Riding was a bit easier each day and horses didn't look like running away with me any more, but I would come back puffing heavily. I ached all over and my back was worst of all. I wasn't getting enough oxygen into my lungs and at times there was no feeling at all in my feet. In those early weeks I was exhausted after riding out. I used to sleep on the lawn in the mornings and go to bed early every night.

Much of the time he would walk round the stable barns barefoot, trying to stimulate some feeling. One day a nail penetrated his foot by fully half an inch but he felt no pain at all, merely slight discomfort. His stay at Camden was also memorable for his first—token—shave since his illness.

It was just a bit of bum fluff really but at least it was a start. The hair grew again on my body first, but it took much longer to appear on my head and face.

Jonathan Sheppard, the only Englishman training in Camden, visited Burly Cocks's barn one morning. "I heard this odd-looking fellow say 'Good morning Jonathan'," he recalls. "I didn't know the man so I nodded in reply and asked Burly the identity of his new work rider. I couldn't believe it when he said it was Bob. I'd known him very well from previous visits but now he looked so awful I didn't recognize him. He looked terrible, pale and light with a little bristle on his head."

In his last week at Camden a horse Bob was riding in fast work crossed his legs and fell, firing his jockey heavily into the ground.

We hit the ground hard and I had quite a few bruises but the thing that pleased me was that I stood straight up. The old man hadn't lost his nerve.

After three weeks in Camden, Bob drove Burly's son, Winky Cocks, on the one-thousand-mile journey to New York where they supervised the stable's two-year-olds for a further week. Bob stayed with his friend Tommy Skiffington. Over the next week Bob rode at least six horses each morning at the Belmont track in New York. His physical progress in that first month in America was considerable. He lost a stone in weight. Much of the excess fat in evidence at Liverpool had melted away. Some of it had been transformed into muscle. The rest had been shed by hard work and constant exercise, as Bob confirms.

When I was first down at Camden my riding muscles were so painful. When I jumped off at the end of a gallop my old legs would almost give way. Though I still ached I was noticeably fitter and, best of all, my hair was growing quite quickly at last. It was much blonder and softer than before but I wasn't complaining.

After a week in New York Bob moved on to Hermitage Farm near Unionville, Pennsylvania, some three hours' drive from New York. The farm, set in delightful countryside, is Burly Cocks's training base for eight months of the year. Bob spent a further week there riding work, playing tennis, swimming and exercising at the health spa in Unionville. Still his feet were a major problem.

Sometimes playing tennis I would have to think in advance before turning. If I did anything quickly I fell over. *You* try running when you can't feel your feet. I used to leave my shoes off when running or playing tennis to try to force some feeling back.

His hands were not right either. The feeling hadn't returned properly. Strength in his fingers was not a problem, but he would drop plastic cups at parties because he couldn't feel them.

Burly Cocks noted Bob's considerable improvement with immense satisfaction. "Everyone at the stable realized how determined he was to ride again and now it was a distinct possibility. We had a talk one morning early in May and he felt he might be ready to ride in a race in another month."

Bob flew back to England on 6th May for his next check up at hospital and a brief holiday at home. The results of the tests were excellent. His blood markers were perfect. His doctors, surprised at his rapid improvement since they had last seen him, were amazed when he told them he planned to ride in a steeplechase in America at the end of the month. Bob spent two weeks in England visiting his family and friends and riding out on most days for Paul Cole, Peter Cundell and, once, Josh Gifford. Jim Old pressed him to consider taking the ride at Newton Abbot on 21st May on Joint Venture, a horse Bob had won several races on in previous years. Jonathan Sheppard rang from America to offer him the plum mount on the brilliant chaser Martie's Anger in a 25,000 dollar race at Hard Scuffle on the same weekend. Martie's Anger had a favourite's chance and if he won Bob's percentage of the prize money would be 2,500 dollars—a considerable sum of money for someone who had been out of work for so long.

Bob turned down both rides for different reasons.

The opportunity to ride Joint Venture was very tempting. I knew the horse well and he had an obvious chance. I looked at the likely runners for the race at the four-day stage and was getting quite excited about it but I was only kidding myself. I was nearly ready but I wanted another week or so to make sure. More importantly, Josh had done so much for me in the past year that I wanted my first ride in England to be for him. Jim understood how I felt. He was a great friend and was trying to help.

Joint Venture, ridden by John Burke, finished a distant third at Newton Abbot. Martie's Anger, however, won at Hard Scuffle, but Bob doesn't regret missing the ride on him.

I thought about Jonathan's offer seriously and rang him back to explain that I was not quite ready. Martie's Anger was too good a horse in too big a race for my comeback. Naturally I didn't want to make a fool of myself first time. I wanted to be sure. I was prepared to try in a small race where I had nothing to lose. I wasn't going to put myself in a major race after such a long lay-off. It wouldn't have been fair to the owners, trainer, punters and even myself.

After months of silence, Bob agreed to talk about his illness and comeback in a full page feature in the *Sunday People* on 18th May. His doctors encouraged him to do so and the response from the paper's readers was instant and heartwarming. Bob received numerous letters of congratulations and support, and several from patients in hospital who had been lifted by his story. As Dr Jane Merrow says, "The article on Bob inspired the other patients considerably and the publicity that followed that initial story affected them all. The patients in hospital only see each other. They are all ill from the treatment, low and pretty fed up. They don't see the people who are cured and generally they don't hear about them. Bob's story was extremely beneficial to the others. It showed if you are determined enough you can overcome the most serious illness."

Bob returned to America on 23rd May expecting to ride Baronial in a steeplechase at Fairhill a few days later, but in his absence the horse had been entered in a more suitable earlier race with a lower weight and had won ridden by John Cushman. "I didn't mind at all," Bob says. "I wasn't in a hurry to come back. Time was on my side."

On Friday, 30th May, Jonathan Sheppard asked Bob to ride a novice chaser, Ripon, at Fairhill the following day. Ripon had been a useful horse on the flat but clearly had his own ideas about jumping fences. He popped over them safely enough in a schooling session on the Friday morning but Bob felt he was not quite fit enough yet to run. There was a second entirely sensible reason for his reluctance to ride Ripon at Fairhill the next day. The horse had turned a somersault at the first fence on his initial outing over jumps and had crashed through the wing of the second fence next time. Hardly the ideal conveyance, Bob reasoned, for such an important comeback ride. Self-preservation came fairly high on his list of priorities at that stage.

Thankful that he had talked Jonathan Sheppard out of running Ripon, Bob joined some friends that evening for a pleasant meal and a few drinks. Imagine his surprise then on his return to the farm late that evening to discover that Jonathan Sheppard wanted him to ride Double Reefed in a flat race at Fairhill the following day.

That was the moment of truth, the time to test everything I'd done in the previous five months. I'd never ridden in a flat race which made it harder, and I discovered I'd have to carry a bit of overweight. I went off to bed in a right state. I was both frightened and excited but still managed to sleep quite well when my heart had stopped pounding.

Bob woke early, as usual, on Saturday 31st May, rode three horses at exercise and set off for the races with Jonathan Sheppard. Fairhill is a small, undulating, grass country racecourse—more like an English jumping course than the traditional flat; left-handed oval American dirt tracks. Jonathan told Bob that Double Reefed had been a useful horse on the flat early in his career but had become a bit sour. He hoped to convert him into a successful hurdler but thought a run against moderate opposition on an unusual grass course might rekindle his interest. "Mind you," he says, "I didn't know that Bob had not ridden in a flat race before. But he'd spent a bit of time sorting Double Reefed out for me at home and he deserved the chance to ride him in a race."

Nervously Bob changed in the jockeys' weighing-room and despite missing breakfast that morning still weighed out at five pounds overweight at 11 stone 1 pound. There was time for a brief scrutiny of the form of his chief rivals.

Deciphering the American form book is a difficult task for European racing fans but by the time Bob strode grim-faced to the paddock he knew the identity of the two most obvious dangers to Double Reefed.

My horse was favourite, but it pleased me that I still thought like a jockey and was prepared to find out the colours of the jockeys riding the other fancied horses. All the other jockeys were professionals. Flat racing to me was a bit of a mystery. I imagined it was like riding work. Clearly they galloped faster than in a steeplechase but I tried not to worry about the difference. After all if you go faster you must stop quicker.

The race, over one mile and five-sixteenths, was just over a circuit of the sharp Fairhill course. At the start Bob, confident of his mount's superior speed and ability, settled Double Reefed in last place tight on the inside rail as the leaders hurtled towards the first narrow, left-handed bend. There, to his surprise and delight, the field drifted wide allowing him to save precious ground as he stayed glued to the rail. Double Reefed, clearly enjoying himself, lobbed along contentedly in last place for half a mile until his jockey asked him to move steadily through on the inside of the pack. On the last bend, three furlongs from home, the leaders wandered wide again allowing Double Reefed to steal even closer and suddenly, for the first time, Bob realized he was going to win.

Until then the idea of winning had not occurred to me. I had gone out expecting to test my reactions and strength. Now I had to think like a jockey again. I was in third place and it seemed just a question of when I wanted to overtake the pair in front of me. I was getting a bit excited by then but I waited another furlong before asking Double Reefed to go on and win his race. The next thing I knew he was trying to duck in behind the front two. He was not keen at all. That was the time to show who was boss. I picked up my stick and hit him hard, just once, on the backside. That put him back on the bridle and he quickened immediately and shot into the lead, going easily, at what is called the sixteenth pole and won with plenty in hand.

I couldn't really believe it was happening. I was blowing hard at the end of the race but not as badly as I had expected. I was chuffed to bits. I'd ridden a winner straight away and that had taken a lot of pressure off me. I thought I was a jockey again . . . and a flat jockey at that!

Bob and Double Reefed returned to a warm reception from the crowd at Fairhill of around ten thousand people. Jonathan Sheppard, naturally, viewed the result with tremendous satisfaction. "The horse was not easy to steer and could be difficult but Bob won rather nicely after riding a waiting race. He rode him quite beautifully. He had never spoken much about his illness. He was, and is, an undemonstrative person. But he was clearly very, very pleased with himself immediately he came back to the unsaddling area. When he dismounted I said 'That's terrific Bob, what a comeback.' Bob thought for a moment and then replied, almost bitterly, 'That treatment they gave me bloody nearly killed me.' "

His fellow jockeys, aware of the long battle against cancer, showed their appreciation of his successful return by throwing the contents of several buckets of cold water over him. Everyone, it seemed, wanted to congratulate him and slap him on the back. Double Reefed was the 357th winner of his career and came four days before his thirty-second birthday. Bob is essentially a private, introspective person. In his moment of supreme triumph he wanted to be alone. He changed quietly, muttered a few polite "thank yous" to well wishers and walked down the racecourse, unrecognized, on his own.

Who can doubt the mixture of emotions he felt as he wandered aimlessly around Fairhill racecourse for the next half an hour?

I had some things to sort out in my mind and wanted to be on my own to try to understand what I had done. I still could not accept that I had won. It was all too much for me. Basically I wanted to hide. My feelings were too intense.

The next few hours are no more than a hazy memory. Bob eventually found his way back to the weighing-room and was led off to the bar for the first of many celebratory drinks with Philippa Winter and Sarah Lomax, both daughters of English racehorse trainers. Later there was time for more drinks back at the farm before a dance that evening near Unionville. At some stage Bob found a few spare minutes to ring his sister and several of his friends at home with the good news. The time difference between Pennsylvania and England is about five hours, but I cannot think of a better reason for being woken up in the middle of the night. Perhaps it was a bad line, more likely it was the celebrations at the other end, certainly I was half asleep, but Bob sounded totally different from his usual quiet self. He talked non-stop in quick sharp phrases, laughed at his own jokes and assured me quite seriously that Lester Piggott could not have given Double Reefed a better ride.

The party finally ended at around four o'clock in the morning, and I understand from Burly Cocks that there were some expensively purchased hangovers in evidence at Hermitage Farm an hour or two later. Burly expected his first lot of horses to be out, as usual, soon after six in the morning but was so dismayed at the state of all his work riders that he cancelled the rest of the day's exercise. Bob, the cause of this disaster, is unrepentant.

Burly was speechless. In the end he sent us all back to bed for the rest of the morning. It was the only time his horses have stayed in their stables all day in the last twenty years.

"Bob's was a hell of a comeback by any standards," says Burly. "The excitement afterwards was just too much for him. In the morning the boys looked so bad I thought it was better for them to rest a little. It was useless giving them orders in the stables. The horses were better off and much safer staying in the barn."

Bob's state of mind that morning may best be explained by the fact that he had forgotten he had rung Mary and some of his friends in England the previous evening. When his beating head had finally improved to critical around lunchtime he dialled once more several numbers in England to pass on the good news again. Later a shoal of cards followed from him with a cryptic and, it must be said, completely ambiguous message saying simply, "I can still do it, Bob."

There is little enough jump racing in America in June. Bob had just one more ride, on Ripon at Monmouth, finished third and returned triumphant to England for his regular hospital check up. His doctors, aware of his success, were deeply impressed at the speed of his recovery and baffled by the apparently healthy state of his lungs.

"To say we were encouraged by his achievement would be a gross understatement," Dr Jane Merrow confirms, "though we were not entirely surprised because he had always been so determined to ride again. But in many competitive walks of life if you are out of action for a long time the chances are that you don't get back. I think perhaps most of all we were impressed by the speed of his recovery. It was a marvellous achievement and one that we very much hoped would encourage other patients."

While he waited for the results of his blood tests Bob popped up to the Pinkham ward to thank Carol, Nicky and Jenny for their active encouragement and support in the darkest months. There was a second, even more serious reason for his visit to the ward. He wanted to show the present patients there that there was hope for the future. What better way than by walking round the ward, offering a quiet word of cheer, while looking absurdly fit, healthy, sun tanned and, it might be added, not a little overweight?

The vast majority of patients who have suffered the agonies of chemotherapy treatment in the Pinkham ward cannot face the anguish of returning there for even the briefest visits. Naturally they do not wish to revive fading memories of the miserable time they spent there. Bob is different.

I realize why the others don't want to go back and I don't blame them at all. But I know how much it would have helped if I had seen an example to encourage me. When you are lying there being sick every five minutes, fearing the worst, it must be a tremendous tonic to see someone who had come through it all looking well and healthy again. I know it would have made a big difference to me especially at the times I was close to giving up. The treatment is still new in England. People don't realize how bad it is. I certainly didn't and if what I've been through can give hope to just one person then I'll be happy.

Bob's blood tests again proved clear. Aware how pleased his doctors were at his recovery he persuaded them to delay the date of his next check up for a few weeks to give him almost two clear months in America. There was time for a three-day visit to Ireland, a trip to the Irish Derby meeting which ended in a monsoon, a brief stay in Tipperary with Tommy and Liz Stack and then early in July he returned once more to America.

After the high peak of his emotional return at Fairhill Bob found it extremely difficult to ride another winner in America. Rides were scarce, his weight a constant problem. Both Burly Cocks and Jonathan Sheppard confess now that they were worried at his constant dieting to keep to a racing weight. "He was certainly losing too much weight too quickly," says Burly. "I think that's why he didn't look too well at times."

Even so Bob continued his daily exercises with renewed zest.

When I look back now I realize I was far from fully fit at Fairhill. I became stronger and heavier each month. Although I wanted to be a hundred and ten per cent fit before I rode in a race, that was impossible since race riding alone can bring you to a peak. At Fairhill on Double Reefed I was more like eighty-five per cent. I suppose I was as fit as any of the boys starting the new season each year after two months' holiday. Sometimes I worried about my lack of wind. I used to kid myself that if it didn't improve I'd have to change my riding style and copy Andy Turnell or some of the flat jockeys who have brilliant balance and perch much higher up a horse's back. Andy's style of riding seems to demand less physical effort and I thought I'd get by like that for a while until my breathing returned.

Early in August the American jump racing circuit moved on for the month to the meeting at Saratoga, which coincided with a major bloodstock sale that attracts buyers from all over the world. Bob started triumphantly with another success on Double Reefed, this time in a valuable novice chase. His percentage of the prize money was 1,600 dollars.

Within a few days of his second triumph on Double Reefed Bob heard the tragic news that Anthony Robinson was dead. Anthony had become ill again soon after the 1980 Cheltenham festival meeting in March but had still insisted on riding Tied Cottage in a race in April—his only mount of the season. A further operation in July had failed to halt the insidious spread of cancer and he had died at his home in England on 2nd August. He was forty-three. Anthony bore a long, painful and distressing illness with commendable courage and stoicism and remained cheerful to the end.

Anthony was a fervent supporter of National Hunt racing. A successful businessman, he rode his own horse, All Glory, to victory at the Cheltenham festival in 1969 and later enjoyed much success with Good Prospect (the horse now owned by Prince Charles) and Artic Ale. Ireland was his second home and he spent every minute of his spare time there, either racing or staying with his great friends Dan and Joan Moore. Argumentative, certainly, and at times abrasive, he shunned publicity and enjoyed nothing more than an evening spent, drink in hand, talking about jump racing. He started off as a distinctly moderate amateur rider but with the encouragement of the Moore family and his own hard work and application became a fully competent jockey. Even so he always gave the impression that the fun of taking part was more important than winning.

Bob was badly shaken by Anthony Robinson's death.

I was very, very sorry to hear the news because he had put up such a tough and prolonged fight and I believed he had been successful in overcoming his illness. He deserved a better fate. The effect on me was shattering. You can't imagine what was going through my mind. Every time someone dies of cancer it frightens me. His death was a very personal thing. It affected me far more than I like to admit.

Welcome visitors to Saratoga were Brough Scott and a brilliant photographer, Gerry Cranham, who had flown over from England to compile a major feature on Bob for *The Sunday Times*. Brough, as we have already explained, had been a major supporter in the months Bob was in hospital, and Gerry, too, had sent messages and a superb photograph of Bob winning an important race at Kempton on Strombolus in happier times. Now the trio spent several hilarious and hectic days boating, water skiing and jet skiing on Lake George, and racing at Saratoga.

"It was a very special story for me," Brough says, "and one that I didn't possibly believe would ever happen. In those days when I used to visit him in hospital the last thing I thought was that he would be riding again. He would lie depressed in bed and we would talk of his plans to be a jockey again but I knew it was all a ludicrous lie. I used to go through the motions of agreeing with him and hope a miracle might happen. But walking away from the hospital and driving home was a pretty dismal experience. Yet here he was, eight months later, healthy, riding winners and with lots of lovely females surrounding him. I can't think of a better story to write than that."

What particularly impressed Brough and Gerry was Bob's eagerness, almost hunger, to ride as many horses each morning as possible. One day at Saratoga he rode eight, each over two miles, and came back at the end of what should have been an exhausting session ready for a game of tennis. That day *was* exceptional—as Bob confirms.

Eight was a quiet day for me. Sometimes I sat on sixteen. It was the only way. The sole reason I'm fit now is because I sat on so many horses each morning. My legs have so much more muscle on them than before my illness and I'm not as fat as I used to be.

Bob rang Josh Gifford who explained he would not have any suitable runners until the end of August. "Bob would call me and say, 'You don't want me yet, do you? I'm just going off to Virginia.' I'd say, 'Have a nice time with her and give her my love.' Obviously there was no need for him to rush back. He was earning a few bob and keeping fit out there. The news of his first winner was fantastic. I thought when I heard he'd ridden a winner on the flat he must have improved!"

So Bob remained at Saratoga for most of August, riding several horses for Jonathan Sheppard and occasional spare mounts for other trainers. He chose the wrong one in a steeplechase, fell on Canadian Regent and watched Wild Sir, the one he rejected, win easily.

I was furious with myself even though I was unhurt. But at least I was pleased to have a nice soft fall. Once, too, I dropped my reins at a fence. I'd never done that before. I was just too clumsy.

Jonathan Sheppard believes Bob was still not a hundred per cent fit at Saratoga. "Although Bob won on Double Reefed for me, the rest of the month there was not good for either of us. There were a couple of times when I wondered if he had done quite as much on a horse as he would have done before he was ill. But that might just have been because my horses didn't run very well. As soon as he was beaten he accepted it and stopped riding. When I saw him six months later in England he told me quietly, 'I'm fit now.' "

Bob's final week at Saratoga was one he would like to forget. First he was fined two hundred dollars by the stewards at the meeting for dropping his hands and stopping riding too soon in a finish. "All I did was put my whip down. I couldn't have won and still finished second," he fumes. On 22nd August, hours before he was due to fly home, he suffered a crashing fall on Cafe Prince. The horse, twice winner of the Colonial Cup, was one of the best chasers in America but this time he jumped like an awkward novice.

The ground was like concrete there and he buried me. I didn't dare be knocked out because I had a plane to catch but I had a hell of a job getting round the course doctor.

Concussed, bruised, with a cut nose and black eye, Bob was driven to Newark to catch a plane to Kennedy Airport for the connection to Heathrow. He was sick several times on the plane and arrived in England battered, depressed and suffering from jet-lag. His achievement in America had been considerable, but he knew he now faced the most important test of all.

Chapter 12

BOB SPENT THE next few days under the intense, dedicated care of Val Ridgeway, the masseuse at Hungerford Squash Club. She worked overtime to ease his tortured muscles and help him recover sufficiently from the effects of his fall to go for two runs with Pete Fisher. Bob was aware that Josh Gifford wanted Roadhead to race at Stratford on Saturday 30th August and he did not intend to miss the ride on one of his favourite horses. In the middle of the week Bob travelled to the hospital and to his relief once more passed his regular tests before returning to Hungerford for more treatment.

Says Val: "He was in a terrible state when he came to me at the start of the week but as usual he was going to ride on the Saturday whatever I thought. He looked deeply bronzed with a nice head of hair again but I think he was still a bit concussed from his fall in America. By the Saturday he was fit enough."

There were three major flat race meetings on 30th August but Bob's much-publicized comeback ensured an unusually large press coverage of the only jump meeting that day; normally it would have been ignored on the sports pages at that time of year. Under a front-page headline HAIL CHAMPION THE WONDER HORSEMAN the *Sporting Life* carried a suitable photograph and a welcome back message.

Roadhead, a safe, reliable jumper who does not mind fast ground, was favourite in most newspapers to win the City of Coventry Handicap Steeplechase despite carrying the severe burden of top weight—12 stone 7 pounds. Bob travelled to the meeting with Jeff King, a tough, forthright jockey whose endless series of risqué jokes helped Bob forget the ordeal ahead. Once at the course Bob tried to hide and ended up pacing the floor anxiously in the jockeys' changing-room.

This was far worse than Fairhill. I was almost unknown out there. Now all the papers were writing about me and there had been bits and pieces on television and radio. I felt tremendous pressure at Stratford and to be honest I was terrified. I walked the course to keep out of the way but kept bumping into people I knew. Once I was in the paddock it was a bit easier. I had a job to do. I talked to the owners but Josh didn't really give me any orders. He just told me to go out and enjoy myself. I think he knew how nervous I felt. I'd won a lot of races on Roadhead before I was ill and thought the world of the horse. He had always been a lovely ride—he was a genuine, honest racehorse—but I had my doubts if he stayed much more than 2½ miles and the distance of the race at Stratford was 2¾ miles.

Cantering uneasily down to the start Bob found himself beside John Francome on Charlie Mouse and was cheered by John's light-hearted banter. "The boys certainly made me feel at home and I appreciated that," Bob said later.

But this time there was not to be a fairytale ending. Roadhead, jumping soundly as usual, ran well, shared the lead at a couple of stages and threatened briefly on the run to the final fence. Lack of a previous race and the huge weight he was carrying proved too much on the run-in and he finished a close fourth behind the winner, So and So, beaten only four lengths.

"I thought I had a chance going to the last but then he blew up," Bob told the delighted owners before going off to change. It had been a painless return on a glorious English summer day.

No-one was more pleased with events than Josh Gifford. "I was absolutely thrilled with the way Bob looked and the ride he gave Roadhead. He did everything right and then the horse tired as we expected."

Three days later, on Tuesday 2nd September, Bob rode again for Josh Gifford, this time at Plumpton. His mount was Toureen, a slow, extremely moderate animal who had finished tailed off last of three at Fontwell a week earlier. Toureen's exalted position as second favourite in the betting at Plumpton owed more to the expertise of his trainer and the emotional support for his jockey than to his own rocky form. Toureen did not jump well, weakened in the closing stages and finished last. Bob returned seriously worried at the clumsy way he had dropped his reins when Toureen hit one of the fences.

> Normally when you jump a fence you slip your reins to the end of the buckle to allow the horse to have freedom of his head. You'll see jockeys who don't slip their reins be pulled out of the saddle when a horse's head pecks towards the ground. This time I slipped my reins all right but then I lost them altogether as I attempted to gather them in. The same thing happened a month earlier in America but I'd never done it before my illness. The trouble was that the feeling in my hands was still not right. Sometimes I had pins and needles. Sometimes I simply couldn't grip things properly.

Urgently he contacted Dr Jane Merrow who reassured him. "It's our fault and a direct result of the treatment you had. The loss of feeling is yet another side effect of the chemotherapy, but your hands should improve as time goes on."

The next few weeks were exasperating for both Josh Gifford and his stable jockey. Under a new Jockey Club edict which, quite rightly, was heavily criticized, trainers were forced to inoculate their horses with an anti-flu jab by a certain date. No one doubted the wisdom of the ruling, merely the timing of it. Many of Josh Gifford's horses were three-quarters fit and ready to run but reluctantly, at the end of August, he inoculated his entire string of horses—with disastrous results. In the next month they reacted so badly that hardly any of them were fit to race and in the ensuing months it became clear that the injections had seriously affected the health and prospects of his stable.

"It knocked my horses sideways. I'm bloody furious about the whole way the Jockey Club organized the new rule. I think we should have had two years' warning, but if not they should at least have told us in the spring of 1980 so that we could have injected the horses before they went out to grass for their summer holidays."

September, then, was a barren month for the Gifford stable. Bob fretted impatiently at home at first, then slipped over to Ireland to stay with a girlfriend for a few days and picked up two spare rides over hurdles at the Galway meeting for the Curragh trainer, Mick O'Toole.

> I hunted both horses round but it made a change and gave me a bit of a holiday. There was no point staying at home because none of Josh's horses were well enough to run. Ireland's a great place to go for a holiday but the trouble is that the people are so hospitable that you need another holiday to recover when you finally stumble back home.

At home Bob waited anxiously for the chance to ride his first winner in England in well over a year. The firm ground and his own fluctuating weight ensured that there were few opportunities to take spare rides for other trainers. He contented himself by riding out each morning for Paul Cole, playing tennis and squash and running regularly with Pete Fisher.

> It was a difficult month. I couldn't wait to start again but Josh's horses were out of action and there were no spares going at all. My weight was far too heavy. The best way to be light is to be race riding every day.

After three weeks Josh decided to run Physicist, a moderate but consistent three-mile chaser, at Fontwell on 23rd September. The horse, significantly, had not yet been inoculated because he would be finished for the season by the deadline set by the Jockey Club.

By a happy coincidence the Fontwell meeting had been chosen as a fund-raising day for the Cancer Research Campaign. Fontwell, a few miles from Bognor Regis in Sussex, is a tight figure-of-eight course which gives the nimble spectator a tremendous insight into the atmosphere and appeal of jump racing. Once more Bob paced the floor of the weighing-room nervously.

> I must have walked round the room three hundred times. I was aware that people were watching me. Since I came back to England all sorts of papers had written stories about my comeback. The pressure to win was enormous.

In the paddock Josh Gifford played down Physicist's chance of winning. He told Bob, "Remember the horse is very short of work at home. Look after him and if you happen to get into a finish only hit him once. He's far from fully wound up yet and I don't want him to have a hard race and to be knocked about."

Physicist started favourite for the race at 6-4, a fraction of a point shorter than the obvious danger, Bold Saint, who had been placed in his previous two outings. Bold Saint's stamina, however, was a little suspect and Bob thought his only chance was that Physicist might outstay him in the final straight of the race over three and a quarter miles and three complete circuits of the course. The other four runners were virtually ignored in the betting and for much of the race Bob was content to sit close behind the leaders on the tight course as Tudor Mystery and Double Action shared the pace-making. Setting out on the final lap Bob gave Physicist a breather on the top bend then made his first decisive move of the race. Physicist quickened down the hill, jumped into the lead past three rivals at the next fence and held a slender advantage over two more jumps.

Then Bold Saint came past me absolutely cruising. I had a peep over my shoulder to see where the rest were and thought I'd finish a clear second. All the way round the final bend I kept hold of my horse's head so he was balanced, and going to the last open ditch, the third from home, I realized Bold Saint hadn't increased his lead any further. I thought if I could keep giving Physicist little breathers we might still have a squeak as long as I could get a bit of momentum going to the last and land running.

Well, we pinged the ditch and the second last, gaining a length each time and going to the last we reduced the gap to a length and were in with a bit of a chance. At that stage I was just hopeful. I was too out of practice to be confident.

Bold Saint and Physicist were clearly tired as they rose at the final fence. Both jumped it well. Bold Saint landed just in front but on the steep, uphill finish Bob Champion produced Physicist on the inside rail with a deft, finely-timed challenge. Even so for one heartstopping moment it seemed Bold Saint would hold on. Then slowly, inexorably, gloriously, Physicist, driven with strength and determination, inched ahead cheered on by the large sun-drenched crowd. His orders momentarily forgotten, Bob wielded his whip powerfully to ensure Physicist did not stop in the final twenty strides. They reached the line first by a desperately hard-fought half length from Bold Saint.

A funnel fully fifty yards long quickly formed at the approach to the winner's enclosure and a tremendous ovation began as soon as Physicist and his smiling jockey appeared. The applause, certainly the loudest ever heard at Fontwell, reached a crescendo as they entered the coveted winner's circle. Bob slid quietly from Physicist's back, gave him an appreciative pat on the neck, politely accepted a warm kiss from a delighted onlooker, gallantly returned the compliment, muttered something unintelligible to the winning owners, ducked under the rail guarding the enclosure and to further loud applause disappeared gratefully into the anonymity of the weighing-room.

It was a terrific reception. You'd think I'd just scored the winning goal in a Cup Final. Josh came running out to greet me with the owners but I was too overcome to say very much. I was most pleased because I wasn't tired. My wind was fine and I was happy that winning the race would take a lot of pressure off me. I hit Physicist once or twice more than I should have done because I was so desperate to win. If I'd been in form and more relaxed I wouldn't have been so hard on him, but Josh didn't seem to mind. He knew I was not usually a whip jockey.

Later over a large glass of orange—yes, orange—in the Fontwell directors' box Bob was overjoyed.

I've waited a long time for this day and can't fully describe how it feels to have done it on one of Josh's horses. His promise to me in hospital to keep my job open as long as I took to recover gave me a reason for living, something to aim at, though there were times when I doubted if I would ever win another race.

Physicist was Bob Champion's first winning ride in England for sixteen and a half months. Physicist also, happily, was Josh Gifford's five hundredth winner as a jump trainer. No wonder he says, "No other success can possibly give me as much pleasure as this. I told everyone, especially Bob, that I didn't fancy Physicist at all so that he wouldn't worry. Actually I thought he had a very good chance because I was sure Bold Saint wouldn't stay."

On the return journey in the car it was suggested to Bob, quite forcibly, that he should stop at a phone box and order some champagne to be put on ice. He smiled in that shy, almost gentle way of his and replied, "I put some in the fridge this morning." Several bottles of champagne later we moved on for a mammoth celebration at the Five Bells in Wickham, where Dottie Channing-Williams had sensibly laid on even more bubbly. If Bob Champion had a hangover the next morning no man ever deserved one more.

Three days after his superb return at Fontwell Bob rode again, this time at the televised Stratford meeting. His mount in the opening novice chase was a promising young horse, Kindly Night, trained by Jimmy James. Bob had schooled the horse earlier in the week and was satisfied with his jumping. John Oaksey, ITV's commentator at Stratford that day, quite naturally spent much time describing Bob's achievement on Physicist. The cameras followed him on Kindly Night for several minutes as the horses circled round at the start while last minute adjustments were made to girths and stirrups.

Racing, at times, is a tough, uncompromising business. Jump racing, in particular, can provide the cruellest twists of fate, one minute sending spirits soaring, the next bringing them tumbling down to the very depths of despair. The run to the first fence in a two mile novice chase at Stratford is short and the course was quite slippery after early morning rain. Kindly Night galloped towards the first fence, slipping on take off and just struggled over, losing several lengths in the process. Worse was to follow. At the very next fence, an open ditch, viewers watched in horror as Kindly Night, who had clearly lost his confidence, slipped once more as he reached the obstacle. His head and chest crashed straight into the yawning ditch and his back legs came thumping over in a spectacular and frightening somersault which sent his hapless jockey into orbit several feet above the fence. When the cameras panned back to the landing side of the fence a few moments later Kindly Night had galloped off unhurt while his jockey lay motionless on the ground surrounded by worried first aid men. Luckily he was merely winded and bruised.

> The horse bounced me into the air and I've seldom gone higher in a fall. I landed on my nose and hand and he landed upside down beside me. I was just winded. I lay there for a minute with all the wind knocked out of me then realized there was nothing wrong so I got up. Then I had to walk all the way back, several hundred yards, which made me mad. The least the racecourse could have done was to give me a lift back!

Two hours later, long after the ITV cameras had stopped filming, Bob limped out painfully to the paddock, jumped purposefully onto Roadhead's back and proceeded to win the Klampenborg Chase with consummate ease. The following Saturday at Chepstow, this time televised by the BBC, he won a novice chase on Earthstopper and fell in the very next race on the strong-pulling, free-running chaser, Right Mingle.

> A fall and a winner on two Saturdays running, that's all part of the job. Both falls had been heavy ones and I was pleased to be in one piece.

Bob Champion's recovery from such a grave illness gained considerable coverage in newspapers both nationally and locally. As a direct result of this he received numerous letters of congratulations and good wishes, the vast majority from people he did not know. One of the most moving letters came at the end of September from Mrs Joyce Lawrence, from Shoreham by Sea, Sussex. She wrote:

> I felt I must thank you for your most encouraging story that appeared in our local paper recently. My son-in-law, Bob Dumbrill, who is 34, is at present in the same hospital. His case is similar to your own and my daughter had really been uplifted by your story. She has found new hope.
> I don't think I have to tell you how ill he is being with the treatment, it is truly heart breaking to those looking on. In fact we

were beginning to fear that the treatment was more likely to kill him than the cancer.

All of us have truly taken heart from your story and those "well-meaning people" who have given us the thumbs down will be shown the article about you as much as possible. No doubt you have had this sort of thing in your own case.

Bob has been a cricketer, footballer and darts player, he adores sport and we were honestly beginning to wonder if he would ever do these things again. Thank goodness now we can really look forward to the future in that direction with more confidence.

Yesterday evening they told us that his latest blood tests showed an improvement which cheered us no end. Thank you once again, from the bottom of my heart, for the hope you have given us all. We wish you a successful career, with a long and healthy life.

Chapter 13

IN THE SECOND week of October Bob came close to riding winners on both sides of the Atlantic. On Wednesday 8th October, at Cheltenham, he won the first two races of the meeting on Lumen and Right Mingle, both trained by Josh Gifford. Quick, accurate jumping was the decisive factor in both cases. Peter Hopkins, the genial owner of Lumen, was full of praise for Bob's handling of his horse. "Although Lumen had won three races for me the previous season Josh had always insisted we would have to wait until Bob was back as he was the only man able to get the horse jumping well. How right he was. That was the first time Lumen has jumped properly throughout a race and Bob could not have given him a better ride."

Early the next morning Bob flew to New York and travelled on to Hermitage Farm, at Unionville. He stayed the night with Burly Cocks, rode out in the morning, then flew back to New York to ride Down First at Belmont Park on Friday afternoon in the Temple Gwathmey, one of America's oldest steeplechases. Down First, owned by Mrs Miles Valentine, had won the race the previous year but Bob's hopes that he might complete a famous double were ruined when the horse broke a blood vessel. Bob flew back to Heathrow overnight and arrived in England in time to drive to Worcester on Saturday where he finished third on Random Leg.

By the middle of the month, Bob was just about the only person who remained unimpressed by his remarkable comeback. Undemonstrative and at times introspective, he was at first faintly embarrassed by the huge amount of publicity devoted to his achievements. When he had first spoken publicly of his illness, in May, it had been with the active encouragement of his doctors; by October he wanted to forget the illness and concentrate instead on what he had always done best—riding over fences. People who pressed him about his return to racing found him surprisingly reticent about his exploits.

> You see the difference is that everyone else had been surprised that I managed to ride again. I'm not. All along I was convinced I would return. Whatever doctors and others told me I was determined to get back to my old way of life . . . and I've done it. That's all I wanted or expected.

Though he did not know it at the time, Bob's resolve to re-establish himself as a top-flight jockey was about to face the sternest test of all. His weight, which had soared alarmingly in the autumn, was already severely restricting the number of horses he could ride. He had been told by Dr Jane Merrow that most patients on a course of chemotherapy eventually put on at least a stone more than their original weight. Sheer survival had seemed more important at the time and so he had not taken the warning seriously. In the middle of October that extra weight threatened to bring his astonishing recovery to an abrupt halt.

In the years before his illness he used to believe he wasted hard and conscientiously to make the correct weight. Now he knew that previously he had merely been playing at slimming. His weight had become a nightmare. The sauna at Hungerford Squash Club became his second home. Each morning he would be waiting impatiently at the door for the proprietor Alan Curtis to open up for business at nine o'clock. Bob would spend an hour or two in the hot, dry box boiling away unwanted pounds, dash to the races, drive back to Hungerford early in the evening and have a second gruelling session in the sauna. Often he would play squash wrapped in several sets of clothes to shed further ounces. On the mornings he rode horses at exercise for Richard Head and Paul Cole at nearby Lambourn, he would still have a brief spell in the sauna whenever time permitted before leaving for the races. The Squash Club became his office for most days of the week. His intake of food dropped dramatically. He would sip a cup of coffee at breakfast, another for lunch, and restrict himself to one meagre meal in the evening when he emerged grey-faced and emaciated from the sauna.

His punishing daily routine in the sauna would have finished lesser men. The wooden benches inside the cramped box are arranged in three levels. At first as he climbed onto the top level, the heat tended to be at least eighty degrees centigrade and he would pour water frequently onto the coals to produce more steam. He has become quite an expert on the subject:

The important trick is to hold your breath when the steam surges round the box. If you can hold your breath long enough until the steam settles you'll be all right.

When he was sufficiently warm he covered himself in baby oil to help him sweat more freely. Gradually, to the dismay of his fellow slimmers, Bob would advance the temperature until it reached as much as a hundred degrees centigrade. As the heat increased, so he moved down to the lower benches until finally, when the atmosphere was almost unbearable,, he would lie on the floor with his head in a bucket of ice-cold water.

By that stage I've already had enough. If I can stay in there for more than an hour I can lose as much as three, sometimes four, pounds. Once you give in and go outside for a break you won't last much longer. You just give up. So I try to last the first time for at least an hour. It's too hot in there to read so it helps to have company but normally I end up on my own. I don't have any option if I want to go on riding. My natural weight now would be around 12 stone 7 pounds.

Sweating was the only way. What else could I do? I didn't want to try pills again as I thought I'd had enough drugs to last a lifetime. Josh said he didn't mind if I settled at 10 stone 12 pounds as my minimum weight but I tried to squeeze a pound or two more off and once did 10 stone 10 at Sandown in October after a hell of a struggle. The trouble is that you have to weigh out with all your riding clothes on plus saddle, girths, stirrups, surcingle and possibly a breastplate and even blinkers. That lot can weigh as much as five pounds. So my actual body weight was down to 10½ stone most of the time, exactly the same as before I was ill. Yet when I rang John Gobourn one night he told me he had put on about two stone although he took exercise every day. That shows how hard it was for me.

Those of us who witnessed his grim daily battle with the scales feared that it might permanently damage his health, but Dr Jane Merrow assured him that the many hours spent in the sauna, though perhaps unwise, were not at all hazardous. In the past the cupboards in Bob's house had been littered with biscuits, sweets, chocolates and other appetizing snacks that he could devour in the evenings he was at home. Now his weight had become such an acute problem that he cleared all the shelves, thus ensuring that he could not succumb to temptation.

Jump jockeys are a gregarious, warm-hearted, happy-go-lucky breed. Much of their enjoyment at riding winners comes from the celebrations that invariably follow with owners, trainers and fellow riders. While the champagne flowed in racecourse bars and sometimes later in restaurants and nightclubs, Bob Champion tended to sip one glass of bitter lemon and toy with a small piece of fish. Often he preferred to return home (via the sauna of course) to avoid the depressing sight of others eating and drinking heartily.

Constant wasting and sweating is both mentally and physically a tiring business and often Bob was exhausted by the end of the day. He, more than anyone else, realized the dangers of sweating too much and ending up too weak to do a horse justice. The greatest jump jockey in the world is completely ineffective if he does not have the strength to help a big, hard-pulling steeplechaser negotiate twenty or so fences. By sheer bloody-minded stubborn refusal to concede defeat to his soaring weight Bob won his own private battle with the scales. That, he argued, was a hazard which he fully understood. Towards the end of October he faced a second, unexpected and much more treacherous threat to the resumption of his career as a leading jockey. It was one which forced him to the very brink of surrender.

After three months of the new season it was clear, as Josh Gifford had feared and predicted, that many of his horses had lost their form as a direct result of the flu jabs ordered by the Jockey Club. Owning racehorses is a massively expensive business and Josh Gifford's owners were used to winning. Some of them, baffled at the poor displays by their horses, wondered if the jockey who had ridden six winners from a limited number of chances, had fully regained all his former skills and strength.

Condemning jockeys is an age-old sport. In times of crisis they are usually the most obvious targets for complaint and invariably the easiest for disposal. During his years with Toby Balding, when he was gaining experience, Bob had been used to censure and criticism, some of it no doubt justified. Now, his confidence already shaken, Bob bitterly resented being blamed though he was fully aware that on occasions he was trying too hard to win.

The first blow fell at Kempton when Bob rode his old ally Roadhead, second favourite in the Charisma Records Gold Cup on 18th October. Roadhead was in his customary position in the lead when he slipped going into the third fence and was passed by most of the field as he scrambled over it like a raw novice. The incident shook the horse's confidence so badly that he failed to recover his poise, jumped awkwardly for the rest of the race and finished nearly last. "I don't know what happened at the fence but he went to pieces afterwards," Bob says. He had won seven races on Roadhead but the owners, significantly, wanted Richard Rowe to ride the horse next time he ran. On the same day, Bob rode a promising young novice Fredo over fences for the first time. Fredo overjumped and fell at the very first fence. The run of bad luck continued. At Cheltenham Earthstopper, again ridden by Bob, carried a five pound penalty for his previous success and was just caught in the final strides by Corrib Prince. At Ascot on 29th October Fredo was much fancied to atone for his Kempton error. But the ground at Ascot was slippery and Fredo was one of several horses in the race that jumped poorly because of the conditions. He finished a distant fifth.

Bob rode his first winner for two weeks at Sandown on 31st October when he and Glamour Show scrambled home in a photo finish over a distance short of the horse's best. Despite that victory he lost the ride on Glamour Show, too. The next day, again at Sandown, he rode Socks for the master of Hickstead, Douglas Bunn. At the fifth fence Socks made a shocking blunder which gave his jockey no chance of staying in the saddle. Richard Rowe took over on Socks next time. This was not, however, too severe a blow for Bob.

Basically I didn't mind losing that one because the horse had always been Richard's ride. He'd won four races on him while I was ill.

A welcome visitor to Sandown that day was Carol, the nursing sister from the Pinkham ward. She watched anxiously as Bob was brought back in the ambulance. Only his ego was hurt, but she was alarmed by his fall. "I'd seen Bob in the parade ring and he looked marvellous but the terrible dangers of jump racing were brought home to me when I saw him carried into the ambulance on a stretcher. It didn't make sense that he had spent a year recovering from cancer to subject himself to that sort of risk. I thought he was quite mad."

Matters did not improve at Newbury on 5th November. Bob began the day by riding Snow Flyer, a brilliant horse who had suffered persistent leg trouble. Josh Gifford's instructions were clear and precise: Bob should settle Snow Flyer behind the other four runners in the first half of the race and so conserve his energy for the finish. The horse's welfare came first.

Imagine Josh's feelings, then, as Snow Flyer, with a breathtaking leap, jumped past his four rivals at the very first fence. By the second fence he had increased his advantage and only Zongalero, struggling several lengths behind was able to stay in touch. So Snow Flyer continued in the lead, jumping and galloping with great zest, until the eleventh fence. There, to his jockey's dismay and his trainer's anger, Snow Flyer failed to take off at all, galloped straight into the fence, somehow remained on his feet but inevitably ejected his jockey in the process. Bob's reception when he eventually returned was distinctly frosty.

Josh moaned a bit and I don't blame him. The owners were obviously unhappy. They were speechless. I tried to explain I didn't deliberately disobey orders. Once Snow Flyer saw daylight at the first fence he was gone and no jockey alive could have held him. There weren't enough runners to cover him up, and he just took off with me. I was in the wrong but I couldn't help it.

Half an hour later Bob rode Moonlight Express. They were in the lead, going well when Moonlight Express overjumped at the fifth last fence and sprawled so badly on landing that he almost fell. Another chance had gone. Bob ended a dismal hour by winning a hurdle race on Lumen but even that victory did not dispel the growing tension.

It seemed as though Lumen would win easily when he galloped into the lead halfway up the finishing straight but he idled in front and many observers in the stands felt that Bob took matters too casually as Palace Dan launched a furious late run on the stands rails. Lumen just held on in a driving finish but both Josh Gifford and the horse's owner Peter Hopkins feared he had been beaten until the result of the photo was announced.

They rushed out to see me with such long faces and didn't believe me when I said I'd won. I was never worried. I only hit Lumen once because he gave me the impression last time at Cheltenham that he didn't like being touched with the whip. I think he had had too much of that in his younger days on the flat. So I sat and suffered and tried to kid him along, and it worked but I know Josh was not very pleased.

On the following Saturday there were three race meetings but Bob did not have a single mount. He stayed at home, depressed, watching racing on television. Publicly he maintained a brave face but privately he was deeply hurt at the unexpected turn of events. Perhaps it had taken rather longer for him to readjust than he or anyone else had imagined? Certainly the results of the inoculations on Josh Gifford's horses had made his comeback infinitely more difficult. Possibly, too, the effects of his grave illness and the chemotherapy treatment had been even more severe on his system than he was prepared to concede. Who can blame him if, at times, there was a scarcely concealed desperation about some of his race riding?

Of course I was desperate. Things could hardly have been worse. After I lost one or two regular mounts I realized I was in trouble. I could see owners and trainers taking the lead and the whole thing snowballing. It made me more determined than ever to prove them all wrong but I wasn't getting the rides to do it and I was completely out of form. Nearly all Josh's horses were wrong at the time. Because I was losing the rides on some of his horses other trainers didn't have the necessary faith to put me up.

On Monday morning, undaunted, Bob rode out at Findon for Josh Gifford and was filmed by Southern Television as part of a feature they were preparing on him. The cameras moved on to Fontwell the same afternoon in time to catch Bob winning a two-and-a-half-mile novice chase on Ta Jette, who was completely unfancied by the stable. Bob Champion excels in novice chases. A natural, gifted horseman with the most sympathetic silken hands, he relishes teaching a young horse to jump properly. When a horse gallops too close to a fence he is able to educate it to shorten its stride and fiddle the obstacle safely; when the opposite occurs and the horse meets a fence perhaps too far away he can ask it to stand right off and jump boldly. The television feature, then, was a success with the added bonus of film of him winning. Despite recent events Josh Gifford, typically, made it clear in an interview that he firmly supported his stable jockey.

But his faith was soon to face its toughest test. Two days later on 12th November Bob rode Fredo again at Newbury. The horse ran a fine race, jumped well throughout but was beaten three lengths by Dom Mancini, whose form over hurdles was infinitely superior. "Bob gave him a good ride and did nothing wrong at all," confirms Josh. At the Ascot weekend meeting several of the stable's horses ridden by Bob ran disappointingly. Random Leg, in particular, ran abysmally.

Josh Gifford was tormented by doubt. "The crime of the whole situation is the damage you are doing when you are running the horses unaware that they are wrong. Random Leg, for instance, had seemed fine at home and appeared to have done well since his last run. The horses in my yard were just like children in a class. The flu spread right through the lot of them. They would run well first time, look well, then run diabolically second time.

"It was all having an effect on Bob. He'd been jocked off one or two and that was worrying him. When he woke up in the morning

I'm sure the first thing on his mind was that he must start riding a few winners.

"I was disappointed with a couple of his rides but it might have been the horses. I can't be sure. Everybody is quick to criticize a jockey. I know because I've ridden. Perhaps he was trying too hard and was relating his anxiety to the horses who were doing too much all through a race. Certainly when he first resumed he was not reading a race as well as he used to. The pace, the run of the race, that sort of thing. In the old days he was content to drop one out if the pace was too hot. Now he was chasing, chasing from the start. That may be because the horse was not going. The flu vaccinations may have caused it."

Josh Gifford, a good sensitive man, was only too aware of Bob's anguish. "I realize that when you start bollocking jockeys you merely deplete their confidence. When my jockeys do something wrong I don't harp on it. Bob wanted encouragement, not the opposite.

"In our good years before his illness I didn't give him any orders. I started off the 1980–81 season in the same way and soon felt the difference. Obviously he had been out of touch for so long that he had become a little rusty and he needed the help of some orders again. When you miss a year and a half you are bound to take a while to regain your feel and confidence. A lot of my horses were new to him. After his illness he was receiving a hell of a lot of publicity and that was putting pressure on him and maybe affecting his riding as well.

"I'm lucky. I have very good owners but some of them understandably wanted Richard because he had won on their horses in the previous season. My owners were marvellous to Bob when he was ill but when it came back to his riding again it was a rather different matter. Owning horses is an expensive hobby. Some of them didn't want Bob on their horses. It was awkward for Richard too. He had done so well in the previous season and was now only sharing the rides."

The crisis deepened on 20th November. Bob had won on both Earthstopper and Glamour Show in previous weeks but was replaced on both of them at Kempton by Richard Rowe. Bob travelled instead to the minor meeting at Towcester and mustered a second place and a third place from three rides for Josh. Back at Kempton both Earthstopper and Glamour Show won. It was a grim time for Bob.

> I knew some people thought I wasn't as good as before my illness. It was obvious to everyone in racing I was getting the elbow, or jocked off as we say. If they thought I didn't have any confidence they were right. It was knocked sideways. I spent hours in the sauna wondering if everything I had worked for had been wasted.
>
> All right. Owners are the ones who pay the bills so they are more than entitled to say who they want to ride their horses. But if I'd been given the choice I'd have gone to Kempton. That was the first time I thought of packing it all in, but I was so upset I wanted to show them I could still do it. The only way to do that was to persevere.

In the middle of this depressing run Bob returned to hospital on 27th November for his first medical check up in two months. In the days leading up to his appointment he worried constantly about the outcome, paced the living-room of his house nervously, and at night found sleep an elusive ambition. He knew that twenty-five per cent of patients with his type of cancer relapsed in the first year after chemotherapy treatment and in his prevailing mood feared that the usual blood tests and X-rays would reveal signs that the cancer had returned.

At the hospital the assistant in the clinic found it quite impossible to put a needle into the vein in his arm to draw off the necessary amount of blood. The sample was taken instead from the back of his hand. Bob comments:

> I know exactly how it must feel to be a pin cushion. One of the nurses in the ward worked out that I must have had about two thousand needles stuck in me during the previous fifteen months. The vein on the inside of my arm was much too hard and fibrosed to take any more needles.

The tests were all clear. His blood markers were perfect and X-rays revealed nothing unusual. Bob popped up to the Pinkham ward to see Carol and Jenny and left for home in a happier frame of mind. It did not last long.

On Sunday 30th November he heard he had lost the mount of Fredo at Folkestone the following day. Bob spent Sunday morning in the sauna and the rest of the day sitting miserably at home in a mood of black despair, unaware of people and conversation around him. His spirits were at their lowest ebb and several times during the long afternoon and evening, when he consented to speak, he insisted that he was going to give up the unequal struggle.

> After this there's no point in going on. Soon the only ride I'll have left will be the trainer's hack. There's no point in going on.

Losing the ride on Fredo undoubtedly hurt Bob Champion hardest of all. The deep wound was open for all to see. The pain was on his face and in his every movement and nothing his cheerful girlfriend Jo Beswick could say seemed remotely like lifting his spirits.

> Well, how would you have felt? I'd come back from the dead and had not expected that sort of thing. I'd been too busy getting fit again to consider it. Racing's a hard game but I couldn't believe what was happening. I had two options. I could pack up there and then, go off to the United States and think about training, or I could stay and fight.
>
> I wasn't sure there was any point in fighting any more. I could see the owners' point of view though I didn't agree with it—the horses weren't winning with Richard either. I couldn't see any sense in going freelance. If I left Josh, who had done all he could do to help, I wasn't going to get many good rides elsewhere.

Ironically Fredo, ridden by Richard Rowe, fell at Folkestone. Two days later on 3rd December Bob travelled to Fontwell hopeful that he might at last ride a winner again, either on a nice young horse Topseed in a novice hurdle or Right Mingle in a long-distance novice chase.

When your luck is out in racing fate can be outrageously unkind. Topseed, going well at the time, turned a somersault at the tight top bend—nowhere near a fence—leaving his jockey dazed, bruised and totally unaware of his surroundings. Clearly concussed and limping badly, Bob was led back to the weighing-room quite unfit to ride again that day. Half an hour later he struggled painfully up the grandstand steps in time to see Right Mingle, ridden in his place by Richard Rowe, come home the easiest of winners.

Bob recovered sufficiently at the weekend to ride two of Josh Gifford's horses, Sweeping Along and Moonlight Express, at Cheltenham. Both finished tailed off behind the other runners.

Chapter 14

DEPRESSED, MISERABLE, HIS confidence at an all-time low, Bob drove on Saturday 13th December to the televised meeting at Ascot where he had three booked rides for Josh Gifford. The week had been a particularly barren one. Frost had caused the loss of Nottingham on the Monday and Plumpton on the Tuesday. When racing resumed, no-one had wanted his services on Wednesday, Thursday or Friday. Bob felt, with some justification, that he had become the forgotten man of racing. His weight was a constant problem, rides were scarce and his stable was right out of form. He had not ridden a winner for five weeks and could not see the prospect of a single success in the days ahead.

Pillager, his first ride at Ascot, did not lift the gloom. A big, slow novice, he led for more than half the distance in the Killiney Novices Chase but was soon passed by more fancied horses when the race began in earnest.

Henry Bishop, Bob's next mount in the valuable SGB Chase, was taking on Venture to Cognac—considered the best young chaser in the country—and two other extremely useful three-mile horses, Doddington Park and Silent Valley. There were only four runners but the best place Bob could possibly hope for was third. During most of the race, Henry Bishop and his disconsolate jockey tracked the other three runners. The final mile at Ascot from the bend at Swinley Bottom is entirely uphill and as stamina came increasingly into play, Bob was delighted and surprised to feel Henry Bishop full of strength and running. He soon closed right up to his rivals, jumped the fourth last a length or so behind the leader Venture to Cognac, then surged to the front with a magnificent leap at the seventeenth fence, the third from home. Urged on by his jockey as

151

he landed, Henry Bishop quickly opened up a six length gap over his pursuers. It seemed the decisive move of the race.

On the long run round the bend into the finishing straight, Henry Bishop maintained his clear advantage and was already being called the winner as he popped neatly over the penultimate obstacle. But then, as he approached the final fence it was obvious he was tiring. Had he made his dash for the winning post too soon? But behind him the others were plainly tiring too—Doddington Park had dropped right out and both Silent Valley and Venture to Cognac seemed to be toiling unavailingly to close the gap. Aware that Henry Bishop was leg weary, Bob held him together at the last fence, made sure he crossed it safely, then drove forward towards the winning post with every aid at his disposal. Bob Champion, in a driving finish, is not perhaps the most tidy jockey in the world, but years of practice had made him a difficult man to beat and now he did not intend to relinquish his hard-won advantage. Venture to Cognac closed the gap substantially but Henry Bishop, though near to exhaustion, held on in an exciting finish by two lengths with Silent Valley a further half a length away third.

Henry Bishop and Bob returned to a hero's reception. Bob's immediate feeling was one of intense relief.

Whatever anyone else thought and said in the previous weeks I knew I could do the job and that win showed it. I hoped it would ease a lot of pressure that had been building up on me.

Thirty-five minutes later Bob strode out with a new spring in his step to ride one of his favourite horses Kybo in the Frogmore Handicap Chase, which offered £4,184 to the winning owner. Kybo was named from the initials of well-meaning messages sent frequently to his owner Isidore Kerman by his mother while he was at school: "Keep Your Bowels Open." An ironic enough name, thought Bob, considering his own prolonged attacks of constipation during his illness.

Kybo had been a brilliant hurdler, good enough to run twice in the Champion Hurdle at Cheltenham. On the second occasion in 1979 he was matching strides with the eventual winner Monksfield when he fell at the second last hurdle. While Bob was ill, Kybo had begun a new career over fences, ridden by Richard Rowe, and had won two of his three races before a suspicion of leg trouble persuaded Josh Gifford to rest him for the remainder of the season. Although Kybo was unbeaten in five races at Ascot, the Frogmore Chase was his first race for thirteen months. He was harshly handicapped, the distance—two miles—was short of his best and his trainer felt he was certain to need a run before he reached his peak.

Josh's orders were simple enough: to look after the horse and enjoy myself. I knew how to ride him. He had so much speed I planned to drop him right out, pick them off one by one and pull him up as soon as he became tired. Everyone was certain he was too unfit to have any chance of winning and looking at him in the paddock I was sure they were right.

Kybo drifted steadily out in the betting and was largely ignored by racecourse punters at 14-1 by the time he set off last of the ten runners. Settled and relaxed at the rear of the field he lobbed contentedly along for the first half-mile fully twenty-five lengths behind the tearaway leader, Siberian Sun. But running down the hill towards Swinley Bottom, a series of breathtaking leaps took him effortlessly past lesser rivals. Turning up the hill with a mile left, Bob thought for the first time that Kybo might possibly win, though he knew he was far more likely to tire rapidly in the holding ground. Waiting patiently, not daring to risk the horse's suspect legs after such a long lay-off, Bob nonetheless found himself making ground steadily on the leaders. Three fences from home Kybo was lying fourth and going best of all, but as he moved up on the bend to challenge the first three, the horse lurched suddenly as he changed his legs. It was the sign that his jockey had most feared: Kybo, it seemed was lame. For a fraction of a second Bob quite seriously considered pulling the horse up because he thought he had broken down badly. The video film of the race clearly shows him check the horse's surging run towards the leaders. Kybo's own matchless competitive spirit made up his jockey's mind for him. The horse found his stride again and was galloping so powerfully and willingly that Bob was only too happy to continue in the race.

In the previous five weeks Bob had forgotten what it was like to ride a winner and had begun to doubt if he would ever experience that heady feeling again. Now he was poised to complete a famous double in successive races. Dramatist, a useful and consistent chaser, forged clear in the straight to such effect that Kybo was the only one able to mount a telling challenge. Dramatist still held a fractional lead going to the final fence but Kybo, in full flight, quickened as only a top class horse can, soared boldly over the fence, landed in front and sprinted up the short run-in to a thrilling victory. Kybo felt unsound again as he pulled up so Bob jumped from his back and led him towards the winner's enclosure with a mixture of emotions.

> Winning that race was the best moment of the season so far. But I wasn't happy at the thought that Kybo had broken down in the process. He was absolutely brilliant and I was beginning to think I might be a jockey again.
>
> As you know I won on both Kybo and Henry Bishop over hurdles before my illness and I always told Josh they would be top class over fences. Today proved that forecast right but I must admit there were times when I wondered if I would be around to ride them. A year ago I was barely able to walk unaided. The whole business of my illness still petrifies me but as far as I was concerned there was no point in living if I couldn't be a jockey.

Happily Kybo seemed to be walking without any hint of lameness by the time he reached the enclosure and no man was more pleased than Josh Gifford to welcome back horse and rider. "Obviously I was delighted for Bob that he had ended such a long sequence in such style. But even more I was thrilled that he had looked after the horse and given him every chance in the first three-quarters of the race before thinking about winning."

Ironically Kybo returned home to Findon perfectly sound while Henry Bishop was found to be lame and could not run again for many months. Even so, Bob's luck had changed with a vengeance. In less than forty minutes he had earned around a thousand pounds from his percentage of two rich prizes. His battle with the scales was, for once, ignored. After a few drinks with Josh Gifford and the delighted owners he moved on to a series of celebrations, first at a wine bar in Windsor and then for a large steak (without chips) at Dottie Channing-Williams' pub where more champagne was already on ice. His delight at crossing so many fences at speed in the afternoon may well explain his attempt to jump a Berkshire hedge in his car late that night on the way to the Five Bells. This time he failed to complete the course for the very good reason that his car was wedged firmly on top of the thick hedge. Luckily help was at hand in the shapely form of Sarah Wickins, a director of British Car Auctions, who gallantly gave him a lift to his rendezvous at the pub.

On Monday morning the *Sporting Chronicle*, above an admiring story, carried a huge headline, CHAMPION THE WONDER JOCKEY. Other newspapers, too, had followed up the story of his Saturday double. If he was impressed by such unstinted praise the next two racing days soon brought him back to reality. At Leicester on Monday and Folkestone on Tuesday he rode a total of four horses for Josh Gifford. None of them ran well.

Back at Findon after racing at Folkestone, pouring outrageously large whiskies, Josh Gifford admitted, "I'm desperate now. Nobody could be more against injecting horses than me. My vets are living in the yard, their bills have gone up from two hundred to eight hundred pounds a month and we still have to find out what's wrong with the horses. The ones that normally would have been winning have finished tailed off, sometimes distressed. As you know I have had my worries about Bob, too, but I'm sure those two winners at Ascot on Saturday will have done his confidence the world of good. I'm perfectly happy with his riding. The horses have not been well enough for him to do himself justice. I'm quite certain his health is fine, but I've been a bit concerned about his weight. Perhaps he's been wasting too hard. I'd be happy if he did eleven stone and just rode the good horses, although it's a difficult thing to do."

On Wednesday evening both Bob and Josh appeared in a televised celebrity showjumping event for charity at Olympia. Bob's team included the three-day-event rider Lucinda Prior-Palmer, nine-year-old junior rider Maria Edgar, and the Olympic runner Beverley Goddard. In a timed contest the riders each had to jump around the course and then the runner sprinted round on her own feet. The winning team was the one with the quickest combined time. Bob completed a fast clear round but his team finished third. A little later the same riders were expected to take part in a camel race. Mark Phillips, Josh Gifford and John Francome were all loaded aboard the ungainly creatures to the considerable amusement of the packed crowd. Bob, perhaps remembering an unhappy experience with a camel at the Newbury Show a few years earlier, was this time conspicuous by his absence.

> I hate the bloody things. They smell, they kick, they bite and it's a hell of a long way down if you fall off. It may look funny when you are riding one but it's not so amusing to be sitting up there feeling like a small boat tossed about in a storm at sea. They make me feel sea-sick so I stayed out of the way in the bar.

Josh Gifford, unsure of his weekend runners, agreed that Bob could go to Towcester on Saturday where he had lined up several promising rides for other trainers. There, for the second successive Saturday, he won two races at a televised meeting. He made all the running on Brown Jock in the three-mile chase and completed an easy double on Acarine in a novice hurdle. In between he came agonizingly close to a third winner on Sea Captain, who led until the final few strides of the novice chase.

> Nothing could stop me by then. I was certain I was riding as well as ever and I think that day proved it. The thing that pleased me most was that both horses were for other stables. Until then all my winners had been on Josh's horses. It showed other trainers were prepared to give me a chance but most important of all the few owners of Josh's who doubted my fitness and strength must have been having second thoughts.

Bob's double at Towcester brought an unexpected bonus a few days before Christmas. A letter from the Racing Information Bureau revealed that he had been nominated for a magnum of Louis Roederer Champagne for his riding that day and he collected it in time for Christmas. In that same week, both Bob Champion and Josh Gifford featured in the annual awards list compiled by the *Sporting*

Life's controversial columnist Jack Logan. Logan elected Bob Jockey of the Year for the courage behind his comeback with all his skill intact. Josh Gifford was named among the Trainers of the Year for his loyalty and compassion in keeping his top stable job open for Bob.

Christmas is a difficult time for jump jockeys. A series of parties including the traditional Jockeys' Dance on 22nd December, leads up to the biggest jump racing programme of the year on Boxing Day. While the rest of the nation settles into an orgy of eating and drinking most jump jockeys tend to pick moodily at spare pieces of turkey. Bob was no exception. He spent a happy, relaxed Christmas day at the Husseys' farm with all the family, including his parents, and sat idly at the table as everyone else gorged themselves on a massive roast turkey with all the usual seasonal trimmings. Early in the evening, as tea was produced, he quietly made his excuses and drove to the sauna at Hungerford Squash Club which had been opened for two hours at his request. There, no fewer than eight jockeys squeezed into the steaming sauna trying to shed the excesses of the previous few days.

Bob spent a further session in the sauna early on the morning of 26th December and his days of self-denial over the holiday were amply rewarded at Huntingdon in the afternoon when he won on Abbey Brig for Josh Gifford. On New Year's Eve he rode in three of the four races at Cheltenham televised by the BBC. His experiences that afternoon illustrated only too vividly the ups and downs in the life of a jump jockey. His first mount Random Leg was still in contention and travelling at a speed in excess of thirty miles an hour when he clipped the top bar of the last hurdle and turned the most horrifying somersault on landing. Bob lay still for a few moments then picked himself up, a little dazed, and ran back to the weighing-room to change for his next ride on Kybo, who duly won the £4,787 Colt Car Diamond Chase as comfortably as expected. Then Bob found time for a breathless interview on television with Julian Wilson. Just over half an hour later he lay groaning on the ground again after a mistake by Pillager at the sixth fence in the novice chase sent him tumbling onto the soggy grass.

"It's all in a day's work," he muttered painfully, nursing a dislocated thumb, as he headed back that night for yet another session in the sauna at Hungerford Squash Club. He had five booked rides at Leicester the following afternoon.

Bob's sixteenth victory of the season on Right Mingle at Leicester on New Year's Day 1981 came exactly a year to the day that he left hospital for the last time. Had he expected his comeback to be such a long, painful and distressing one?

Not really. Though I didn't know what to expect. The weight was one problem that I didn't anticipate. But perhaps I was a bit naïve to imagine that all the owners would want me back on their horses straight away. I had to prove myself again and it took a lot longer than I thought because our horses were wrong.

The month up to the middle of December was the hardest of all to bear. I was more upset in that month than throughout the year of my treatment. I was beginning to feel a bit of an outcast. Even so, if I had known how hard it was going to be to re-establish myself I'd still have gone on. Why? Because I like it so much. Racing is my life.

Chapter 15

BOB CHAMPION'S INSPIRING and successful battle to return to such a demanding sport gained its due recognition on 2nd January when a panel of leading racing journalists voted him Amoco National Hunt Jockey of the Month for December. His prize included one hundred gallons of petrol and an inscribed whip. Bob is invariably embarrassed by such awards but even he could not conceal his profound delight at the news when he arrived at Newbury races that day.

It meant more to me than anything I'd ever won, perhaps because the idea of winning it had seemed so impossible three weeks earlier. I was touched all right, but I knew I couldn't have done it without the constant support of Carol and Jenny when I was in hospital, and Josh and all the other people who helped me get back. They kept me going when I was ready to give up.

Bob's good humour did not last for long. In the very first race, a three-mile novice chase, he looked certain to win on the bold-jumping Another Duke until the horse misjudged the last ditch completely, turned sideways as he crashed through it and fell heavily, kicking his jockey in the head and then rolling on his legs. Bob returned pale-faced and shaken, yet determined to ride Ross du Vin in a later race over fences. He sat in the weighing-room looking increasingly ill and eventually agreed, after a bitter argument, that he was not fit to partner the horse. How fortunate. Poor Bill Smith, who deputized for him, suffered a crunching fall at the very same fence that had claimed Another Duke.

Badly bruised and perhaps a little concussed, Bob turned to the faithful Val Ridgeway at Hungerford Squash Club to help him recover in time for the next day's racing. Sure enough, against the advice of well-meaning friends, he rode again the following day, without mishap. No-one could possibly doubt his courage, spirit, or commitment.

The following week Bob learned that his brave battle against cancer had gained him a valuable sponsorship deal with British Car Auctions. Sarah Wickins, undeterred by the sight of his unconventional steering in the lanes of Berkshire three weeks earlier, had proposed that her company present him with a Vauxhall Royale car for the ten months of the racing season. The deal had been suggested by Josie Nicholson, a friend of Bob's and business manager to several sportsmen including the brilliant flat-race jockey, Pat Eddery. British Car Auctions donated the car to Bob and paid the tax and insurance. He merely had to drive it and fill it with petrol— which was not a problem since he had just won a hundred gallons. Bob visited the company's offices, had lunch with several of the directors and drove away contentedly in his smart new car.

British Car Auctions had run a "We Support Sport" campaign for several years, but Bob was the first jockey to join their sponsorship programme. "We admire the courage of all steeplechase riders," Sarah explains, "and were particularly proud to be associated with Bob Champion who had won such a brave battle to return to brilliant racing form. He earned our support by the courage and determination he showed to succeed after such a grave setback." Sarah's father, David Wickins, the guiding hand behind the success of British Car Auctions, was in complete agreement with the deal. He had been a racehorse owner for many years and particularly enjoyed watching his jumpers in action.

A major milestone in Bob's remarkable recovery from the effects of the chemotherapy treatment came on 15th January when he felt confident enough to have his hair cut properly for the first time since his illness. He chose a barber's shop in Newbury. Until January he had been content to allow one of his girlfriends to trim his hair occasionally, but by this time it had become so thick, long and curly that a haircut was an urgent priority.

His racing fortunes continued to fluctuate. On successive days he dislocated his thumb twice more in falls from Moonlight

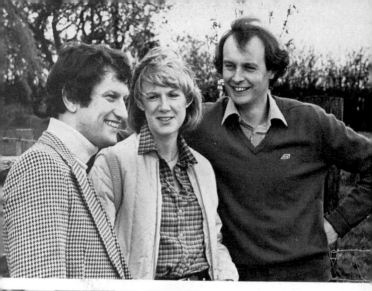

Bob and his wife Jo with
Jonathan Powell.

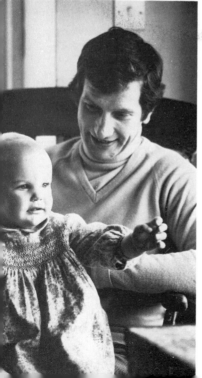

Bob with his
goddaughter,
Lydia Powell.

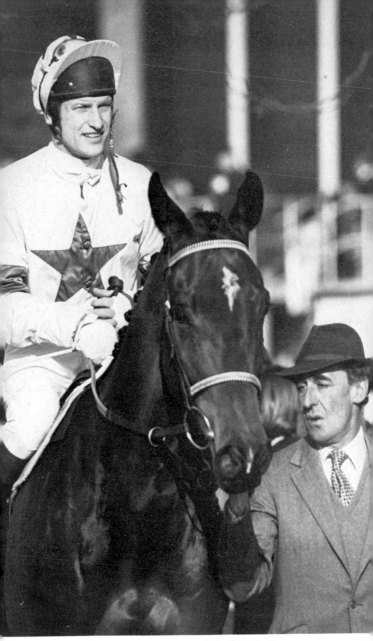

Bob Champion and Josh Gifford.

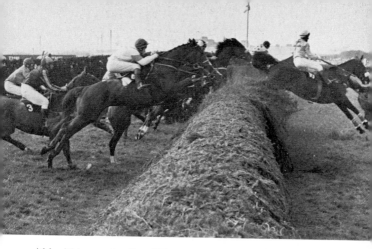

Aldaniti jumps the Canal Turn first time magnificently, with
Spartan Missile (3) the eventual second, just behind.

The village of Findon crowds into Josh Gifford's yard to
welcome the National heroes home.

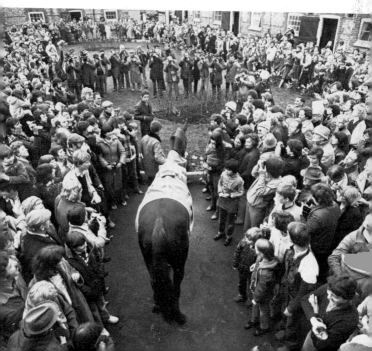

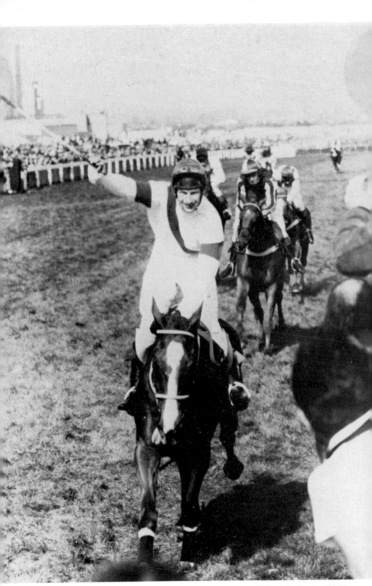

Bob raises his arm in triumph as he and Aldaniti win the 1981
Grand National.

Express and Corbiere. Regular treatment from Val Ridgeway ensured he was able to continue riding, but his thumb was becoming increasingly painful.

The following Saturday was a day Bob describes as the most unbearable since his illness. At Ascot he fell twice more, from Right Mingle and Kybo. Right Mingle galloped off unscathed but poor Kybo had to be destroyed after a heart-breaking accident. He had been going as well as anything in the Jock Scott Handicap Chase until he slipped on landing at the water, did the splits and dropped right out of contention. Bob's first inclination was to pull him up but the horse seemed unharmed so he decided to pop him over two or three fences on the way back to restore his confidence.

Kybo cleared those extra fences with ease but just as his jockey was pulling him up at the entrance to the straight, the horse's near hind leg shattered above the hock. The sudden break caused Kybo to fall to the ground, throwing his jockey over the running rail as he did so. The horse struggled bravely to his feet, limped a hundred yards or so across to the hurdle track and collapsed again where he was swiftly and painlessly destroyed.

Bob, aware of what had happened, climbed dejectedly back over the running rail onto the course, ran to Kybo and gently removed the saddle and bridle from his old friend. Deeply shaken and upset he walked back towards the stands and passed Josh Gifford running down the course to reach Kybo. The distress in the eyes of both men was such that they continued their separate journeys without speaking.

When he discovered Kybo was dead Josh Gifford was so distraught he left the course immediately. Bob, too, was inconsolable.

Why does it always happen to the best horses? They are always the ones who are killed. Kybo was such a brave honest horse, the best I've ever ridden. He's irreplaceable. I know how Josh and the owners will be feeling. I wish I'd pulled him up immediately after jumping the water even though the racecourse vet says it wouldn't have made any difference. He told me the horse must have broken the leg landing over the water and it had been held together for another minute by skin and muscle.

That terrible day contained one more bitter blow. As Bob was leaving Ascot races he heard that Dr Alun Thomas, his specialist in London, had died the previous day.

> That man saved my life. He understood my problem at once. If he hadn't sent me along to hospital that day I contacted him I wouldn't be here now. Alun patched up hundreds of jockeys over the years and we will never be able to replace him. Never. Most of all he was a loyal friend.

Josh Gifford rang Bob Champion on Saturday night and the two men talked poignantly about what might have been. People who imagine that horse racing is mere animated roulette might be surprised at the depth of feeling that a particular horse can engender. Kybo's death was a tragic loss to his owners, trainer, jockey and devoted lad Mark Dixon, who had looked after him for four years. On Sunday morning, soon after dawn, Josh was in the yard pacing miserably outside Kybo's empty box.

After a dismal weekend there was little time for Bob to think of the past. 22nd January proved a notable day. He won on Joint Venture, trained by his great friend Jim Old, and was booked for speeding in excess of ninety miles an hour on the motorway on the journey home. At Newton Abbot Joint Venture, at the age of twelve, stayed on strongly for a comfortable success in a £3,000 chase. It was exactly seven years since Bob had jumped from the horse's back after his first run at Windsor and predicted that he would win a lot of races. How right he was. Joint Venture's success at Newton Abbot was the fourteenth of his career and he had also been placed many times. Says Jim, "Bobby was so keen on Joint Venture in those early days that we nicknamed the horse 'Gold Cup'. I was thrilled that he had ridden a winner for me again. He seemed to me to have been riding better than ever all season and several months earlier I had determined to use him whenever possible."

Late in January 1981 Bob received a marvellous letter from Geoff Moorhouse, father of a young patient who had recovered from the same type of cancer. It read:

I am writing to tell you that my son Colin, aged 22, has just started work again in Arizona after several treatments of chemotherapy and prolonged radiation at the hospital in South London that treated you.

The reason I am writing to you is that *you* did a great deal to get Colin through the chemotherapy; you made him fight the illness. You gave him something to work for during the illness, you Bob Champion were *his hero*.

After his first course of chemotherapy he was so depressed that he was reluctant to fight. The nursing staff in the Pinkham ward gave him a copy of a *Sunday People* article of your remarkable fight against cancer. Colin showed it to me when my wife and I visited him and his words were, 'If Bob Champion can do it so can I.' From that day forth he fought as you did. For all this, from the bottom of my and my wife's heart I thank you one hell of a lot for your inspiring my son. We, as a family, owe you a great deal.

Because Colin read your story and others that followed it, he decided to do one for the local paper here in Hatfield to encourage others to fight. We always look out for your mounts and to see how you are faring and we have even had a bet or two on you. One day Colin and I would love to meet you personally to thank you.

Once again Bob Champion, thanks for what you have done for Colin and us and probably for a lot of other people. Above all, we must thank the nursing staff at the hospital who were terrific to Colin and us as parents.

Yours sincerely,
Geoff Moorhouse

P.S. All my life I shall be thankful to you and the hospital.

On Tuesday 4th February the church of St Mary's in Bryanston Square, London, was packed with mourners for the memorial service for Dr Alun Thomas. Many ex-jockeys were there, including Brough Scott, John Oaksey and Terry Biddlecombe. Numerous other sportsmen who attended the service included the former England cricket captain Mike Brearley and representatives of the Arsenal football team. Bob Champion was not among them.

I wanted very much to be there but I had to go to Leicester for Josh for three rides and one of them won. I think Alun would have understood my feelings. I'm sure he would much have preferred me to win a race than to sit with a long face mourning him. He found enormous satisfaction in enabling his patients to overcome sickness and injury.

The address in St Mary's was given with much dignity by the Royal jockey Bill Smith whose career had been saved by Alun Thomas after he had shattered his knee in a fall. Bill spoke movingly of Alun, the trusted counsellor of jockeys whose clinic had long been accepted as a happy meeting place where aching joints, cracked bones and low spirits could all receive the treatment they needed.

Early in February Bob drove to hospital in London to undertake a demanding series of tests to determine the exact state of his lung function. His doctors were so intrigued by his continuing success that they wanted to assess just how much his lungs had recovered from the damaging effects of the chemotherapy treatment. Fog hung over the M4 that morning like a ghostly blanket. The traffic trickled towards London at a crawl, then stopped several miles from the Chiswick flyover. Restless at first, then downright impatient that he might miss such a vital examination, Bob drove urgently up the hard shoulder of the motorway until he was stopped and booked by a patrol car which had followed him.

He reached the hospital an hour late close to boiling point, and spent the next three hours working off his frustration and anger on a series of exhaustive tests. Initially he was placed in a sealed container, with wires and electrodes attached to his chest to monitor his heart and lungs and he was required to suck and blow into various tubes. Later he moved on to a treadmill which speeded up every few minutes.

At first it was easy although I was wearing all sorts of apparatus, including a big heavy mask on my face. Gradually you are forced to walk steeper and steeper uphill as the treadmill is speeded up. Every three minutes it moves up a gradient. In the end you are walking as fast as you possibly can without running. I was on the machine for twenty minutes which was a record for someone who had six chemotherapy treatments. They told me to ring a bell when I was too tired to carry on but the only reason I stopped was because I was bored and the weight of the mask on my head was proving too much.

He also gave samples of blood from his ear lobe at the start of the tests and again when he was tired at the end.

I was quite pleased with myself for once. Considering I'd had eleven falls in the past month I thought I was extremely fit, probably stronger than I'd ever been before my illness. The tests proved to me that my wind was as good as ever.

Three days later he received a most encouraging report from the hospital specialist, who wrote:

When we last tested you, a year ago, your lung function was moderately impaired because of the bleomycin. This time there has been a very substantial and pleasing improvement such that your lung volumes are normal again and gas transfer is around the lower limit of normal. Moreover, at exercise you were able to do more than almost anyone we've ever tested and even at this high level of exercise the lungs were able to keep the blood fully saturated with oxygen, which is a strong pointer to normal lung function. We can say you have very little residual lung damage indeed from the bleomycin which is pleasing to us too.

One of the assistants told us you gave him three tips but he could not get to the street to go to the betting shop because he was too busy. Imagine how he felt when he heard that two had won and the other horse was second.

The second week of February was a momentous one even by Bob's high flying standards. On Monday 9th February he won on Another Duke at Fontwell and travelled on with fifteen other jockeys to a boxing dinner in their honour at the Anglo American Sporting Club in the depths of the Hilton Hotel in Park Lane. Imagine his surprise and embarrassment when he reached the hotel to discover that he alone was the guest of honour at a function attended by some thousand dinner-jacketed boxing fans. The other jockeys were there strictly in a supporting role.

After dinner Derek Thompson, who had recently moved from BBC radio to ITV, made an amusing and at times emotional speech as he proposed the toast to Bob Champion. John Oaksey, the chairman for the evening, spoke in glowing terms of Bob's recovery before presenting him with a handsome cut-glass decanter together with six glasses. Bob was overwhelmed by the occasion. He rose unsteadily to his feet, mumbled a few "thank yous" and revealed that the first he had known about his being guest of honour was when he saw his name on the front of the menu. He spoke for a few moments more, confessed he was utterly speechless and sat down to thunderous applause. Later he recovered sufficiently to give Derek a lucid interview for a programme ITV was planning to transmit on him the next evening.

An entire table at the dinner was taken over by Derek Thompson's family, including his father, his brother Howard and their friends from Teesside who had come down for the evening. Later the party moved on for further celebrations. Bob Champion finally returned home sometime after four a.m. and discovered in the morning that he had put on no less than nine pounds during the night's festivities. At least he did not have to ride that day and after an exceptionally punishing session in the sauna was fast asleep in bed, like most of the nation, when ITV's feature on him began, with spectacular mistiming, shortly before 11.45 p.m.

On Wednesday Bob set off in relaxed mood for Ascot where he was due to ride Aldaniti who seemed to have fully recovered from the serious leg injury he had sustained at Sandown in November 1979. Aldaniti had certainly suffered more than his share of injuries and training setbacks which had restricted him to only sixteen races over fences. But he had always possessed considerable talent and had finished third in the 1979 Cheltenham Gold Cup and second in the Scottish Grand National a month later. Aldaniti had spent most of 1980 recuperating at the Sussex home of his owners. He had been given a thorough preparation with many weeks of tedious roadwork, first walking and later trotting, usually ridden by Valda Embiricos, before returning into training at Findon shortly before

Christmas for more serious exercise. In the paddock at Ascot he looked well but a trifle burly and his front legs were heavily bandaged as a precaution against further damage.

Josh Gifford and Nick Embiricos did not need to give Bob any instructions. All three knew that Aldaniti's legs were suspect and that he required the gentlest of introductions if he was to have any chance of remaining sound long enough to run in the Grand National early in April. Eight runners lined up at Ascot for the televised Whitbread Trial Handicap Chase, worth £7,596, and Aldaniti started the longest price of all at 14-1 though a few intrepid punters had availed themselves of the 33-1 offered earlier that morning.

Aldaniti, jumping immaculately, settled at the rear of the field which was soon reduced to five by the falls of Lesley Ann, Bueche Giorod and Master Spy. Entering the final mile the front-running pair Cabar Feidh and Royal Charley had established a useful lead and it was clear that Aldaniti, gaining ground at every fence, was the only other runner capable of making a race of it. Bob Champion delayed his challenge as long as he dared in order to give his mount the easiest possible race. When he did ask Aldaniti to go on and win, the response was immediate and electrifying. Aldaniti closed the gap effortlessly, surged into the lead with another fine leap at the second last fence and though hard held by his jockey, kept on strongly to beat Royal Charley by four lengths.

Nick and Valda Embiricos and Josh dashed out to greet horse and rider on the long walk back to the winner's enclosure. Josh Gifford was ecstatic. "Nobody, I repeat nobody, has ever given a horse a better ride than that. I'm not saying it just because he won. Bob looked after the horse all the way, got him nicely settled and jumping and produced him so sweetly that the horse didn't know he'd had a race. I'm thrilled to bits with Aldaniti and Bob. After that I'm not bothered if he runs again before the National. The next seventy-two hours will be decisive. If his legs are still sound after that we are in business. This win has given me more pleasure than you can imagine."

Nick Embiricos, too, was jubilant. A few days later he wrote to Bob, "I was overjoyed by Aldaniti's win at Ascot and have still not really come down to earth after the happiest and most thrilling sporting occasion of my life. Hearty congratulations and all my thanks for giving the horse such a brilliant ride. We saw it all again on Josh's video later and it was marvellous."

Bob Champion, typically, dismisses such extravagant praise.

Riding the good horses is the easy thing about our job. Aldaniti has so much class he was always in a different gear to the others. He's one of the bravest horses I've sat on. He'd keep galloping until he dropped. At Ascot I was merely a passenger.

Early on Thursday morning Bob was just setting off to school a horse for Jim Old in Dorset before going to Wincanton races when Josh Gifford rang to say he would have to go to Huntingdon instead that afternoon. Richard Rowe, who had hurt his ankle on the Monday, was still unfit to ride. Cursing the lateness of the switch Bob barely had time to shed half a pound at the Hungerford sauna before he set off on the long drive to Huntingdon. His first mount there was Rajmataj, handicapped on the minimum mark of ten stone. Bob weighed out at 11 stone 1 pound, no less than fifteen pounds overweight, and finished nearly last.

His humour, however, improved thirty-five minutes later when he was re-united, in the £4,142 Sidney Banks Memorial Hurdle with Glamour Show, the horse on which he had been replaced earlier in the season by Richard Rowe. The irony of the situation was not lost on Bob who, riding like a man inspired, lifted Glamour Show first past the winning post in a triple photo finish. Brown Rose, the horse he was scheduled to ride at Wincanton, fell at halfway and his jockey Steve Knight broke his arm as he crashed to the ground.

Chapter 16

ALDANITI'S TRIUMPH AT Ascot led to a poignant letter to the *Sporting Life* from Mike Lawrence of Harrow, Middlesex. He wrote:

> I was a regular racegoer, hardly missing a Saturday, until, because of a football accident, I had a stroke last November. I am only twenty-four and from leading a very active life am finding it hard to adjust to what may be a lesser existence.
>
> Aldaniti and Bob Champion's recent victory at Ascot gave me great heart. They were both, at one time, very ill but thankfully have now returned to the top. They have become shining examples to me and, through you, I should like to thank them both. It was the most magnificent tonic.

Nick Embiricos was so touched by the letter that he arranged for a photograph of Aldaniti, signed by Josh Gifford and Bob Champion, to be sent to Mike Lawrence.

The same week Bob heard the sad news that Bob Dumbrill, who had also been a patient in the Pinkham ward, had died suddenly and unexpectedly from his illness at the age of thirty-four. Only four months earlier his mother-in-law Mrs Joyce Lawrence had written thanking Bob Champion for his encouragement and support. In February, despite her grief, she wrote thanking him once more:

> There is no doubt that your experiences as told in several newspapers helped poor Bob and his wife. In fact my daughter pinned them on her wall so that whenever she felt despair she was reminded that you had won through. For us it was not to be, but the successes must be made known and if necessary shouted from

the roof tops. My son-in-law was unlucky. Right until the end his optimism remained the same and his courage never wavered. We are just grateful for the chance of life the treatment offered and for encouragement given by people such as you.

The word cancer still terrifies so many people and they don't seek the help they should even when they have the symptoms. The thought of treatment still frightens them. Your experiences, I'm sure, will give encouragement. My family and I have watched your progress with great pleasure.

That kind letter from Mrs Lawrence had a profound effect on Bob Champion and his solemn mood was not helped by the bitterly cold spell that wiped out all racing in England that weekend. He had been due to ride on Saturday at Newbury. The decision to abandon the meeting was a formality so he dashed to Heathrow, heard on the ten-thirty news that Newbury was off and had time to spare to catch the eleven o'clock flight to Dublin with Peter Hopkins, owner of several horses trained by Josh Gifford and another trained in Ireland by the incomparable Mick O'Toole.

At Dublin airport they found a taxi to take them to Leopardstown racecourse on the edge of the city, reached the track in time for the first race and later met Mick O'Toole who offered Bob the ride on Yellow Brass in the richly sponsored Erin Foods Hurdle, the main race of the day. He had just enough time to change into some borrowed riding clothes before rushing to the paddock for the start of the long preliminaries. Yellow Brass led for the first half mile, dropped out of contention when the pace quickened and ran on well again to finish in the middle of the field.

Peter and Bob stayed with the O'Toole family overnight and arrived home to find England still in the icy grip of the cold weather. Newton Abbot, however, on the coast in Devon, was able to go ahead with its fixture on Tuesday and Bob rode another winner for Jim Old there on Intinto. He also feared he had broken his left arm after an ugly fall from Right Regal sent him crashing straight into the solid running rail. Jim bandaged the arm in Animalintex (usually used for poulticing horses' legs) and Bob drove himself painfully home. Luckily the arm was only severely bruised and after several sessions of treatment from Val Ridgeway he was fit to ride again at Lingfield at the end of the week, though the arm was still heavily bruised and painful.

On Saturday Bob took his regular girlfriend Jo, blonde and lively, to the Jockeys' Cricket Team annual dinner and dance at the Frogmill Hotel, near Andoversford in the heart of the Cotswolds. As we ate, danced and drank our way through the night various warnings from the local police about snow hazards were greeted by a mixture of ribald laughter and downright disbelief.

Four or five inches of snow lying on the roads in the vicinity of Andoversford proved a sobering reality at around three o'clock on Sunday morning as we joined some of the early leavers at the start of the optimistic homeward journey. The redoubtable Bob Champion, whose efforts to maintain his bulky frame at a racing weight had as usual precluded such normal activities as eating and drinking, emerged hollow-cheeked to demonstrate at the driving wheel some of the single-minded determination that had helped overcome his grave illness a year earlier.

Andoversford is surrounded by hills. Whichever way we turned in the blizzard our path was blocked. Undaunted, Bob examined his map and set off along a cart track. Denied yet again on that unlikely route and hemmed in by snowdrifts on all sides he headed, more hopeful than confident by now, for the wilds of Bibury, until we encountered yet another steep hill. While Bob stayed at the wheel the rest of us scrambled knee deep into snow and formed the parody of a front row of a dishevelled rugby scrum that, mercifully, was witnessed only by a lone marauding owl. Pushing, slipping, cursing, somehow we manhandled the car up the long, steep gradient until we reached a vast, silent snowbound plateau. The rest of the journey on the icy roads was relatively simple. Some of the revellers, however, remained holed up at the Frogmill Hotel for several days.

Luckily Bob Champion was not among them for he was about to commence the most consistently successful week of the season. On Monday at Fontwell, in atrociously heavy going, his first ride was on Random Leg, the total outsider at 33-1 in a talented field of six for the £6,000 National Spirit Pattern Hurdle. Josh Gifford had wondered about the wisdom of running the horse who would have met his rivals on much better terms in a handicap. "When I woke up this morning I thought I must be crackers to run him at all," he confessed. His anxiety was unnecessary. Bob Champion and Random Leg set out to make all the running, increased the tempo on the second circuit and together galloped gaily home many lengths clear of their mud-spattered pursuers. Eddie, Bob's only other ride of the day, was an equally easy winner of a novice hurdle. Bob continued in form on Tuesday by riding Imperium, trained by Jim Old, to victory in the first race at Huntingdon, completed yet another double on Socks later in the afternoon and came back in a temper convinced he should have won three races after being beaten a short head on Abbey Brig.

I was murdered wherever I tried to go on Abbey Brig. And by a woman jockey. They shouldn't be let loose on a racecourse!

He ended a momentous day with a fall from Scrumping in the novice chase. Frost caused the loss of racing on Wednesday but even the weather could not halt Bob Champion's spectacular progress through the second half of February. The frost lifted overnight, racing was possible at Lingfield on Thursday and for the third time in three racing days Bob Champion achieved a double. He won the valuable Surrey Novices Chase on Earthstopper and the last race on Intinto, his only two rides of the day. Earthstopper, trained by Josh Gifford, was running over fences for the first time. Jumping brilliantly, he led for most of the way, was headed by the odds-on favourite Prayukta in the home straight, but ran on again so strongly that he regained the initiative at the last fence and won decisively. In contrast Bob needed all his considerable strength and determination to force Intinto into the lead in the last stride in a triple photo finish at the end of a competitive novice hurdle.

On Friday Bob did not have a single ride but he travelled to Kempton races anyway because he could not bear to be on his own. Despite his continuing run of success he was unable to sleep at night. Sheer naked fear at the possible outcome of the full-scale medical test he faced the following week occupied his mind at all times. In addition to the usual blood tests and X-rays on the Thursday he was due to have an exhaustive scan two days earlier that would prove conclusively if his body was still clear of cancer.

When you are in the middle of the sort of lucky run I was having you almost expect it to end in disaster. I was terrified at the thought of the tests, far more nervous than at any of the previous examinations. I hadn't had a full body scan since I left hospital fourteen months earlier. I felt well in myself but that was no guide at all since I'd never felt better in my life when I was told I had cancer. Whatever anyone said to me I was still worried. The news that Bob Dumbrill had died didn't help. In those last few days before the tests I became more and more nervous.

After a day's break his winning run resumed unabated. He had two rides at Kempton on the Saturday for Josh Gifford. Both were on television. Shady Deal, his first mount, started at 9-1 in the £3,000 Portlane Handicap Chase, led soon after halfway and kept on resolutely to win by twenty lengths. Shady Deal was Bob Champion's seventh winner from nine rides in the week. An hour later Bob completed a supremely successful week's work by finishing second on Royal Judgement in the feature race of the day, the Tote Pattern Chase.

Bob Champion's earnings for the week from riding fees and winning percentages amounted to almost two thousand pounds. He did not feel like celebrating, however. The tension of his forthcoming tests increased over the weekend and his girlfriend Jo bore the brunt of his bad temper as he became more irritable and grumpy.

> I was horrible because I couldn't stand the strain of those last few days. It's not easy to be nice and calm and pleasant when you are wondering all the time if you'll be back in hospital close to death in a few weeks.

Bob stayed with Derek Thompson in London on Monday night and drove to the Royal Marsden hospital early on Tuesday morning for the most vital tests since his illness. He was noticeably subdued.

> I hate it every time I go back. About two miles from the hospital I can smell that horrible mixture of platinum and sweat. The nearer we get to the hospital the worse the smell. It's the same for other patients. They never forget that dreadful smell. Just thinking about it makes me feel sick.

The most comprehensive body scan took almost two hours to complete. Bob lay unmoving in a long enclosed tube with his head outside, while numerous minute X-rays were taken from one end of his body to the other. Every twenty seconds he held his breath while another X-ray was taken.

Bob had been due to ride at Plumpton in the afternoon but the meeting was abandoned because the course was waterlogged, so he popped up to see the nurses in the Pinkham ward before driving home tired and anxious. He was too worried to sleep that night and was up before dawn in plenty of time to ride out for Richard Head at Lambourn. Much of the rest of Wednesday he spent waiting nervously at home between visits to the sauna at Hungerford.

Early on Thursday, after another restless night, Bob drove back to the hospital for his regular X-rays and blood tests, taken this time from the back of his wrist. Dr Jane Merrow, who is usually in attendance on such days, was able to pass on the good news that the body scan had confirmed that he was completely clear of cancer.

I was totally relieved. I think I smiled for the first time in a week. Dr Merrow said I had nothing to worry about and that I need not return for my next tests for another three months.

There was time for a drink with Carol, the nursing sister from the Pinkham ward, and another with Derek Thompson. When Bob returned home a message on his Ansafone gave him double cause for celebration. John Watt had rung to say he had been voted Amoco Jockey of the Month for February in addition to his December award.

Twice in three months! I couldn't believe it. I thought at first someone was pulling my leg. I never imagined I'd be chosen again which made it all the nicer to win.

Even so, in a month hit hard by the weather, Bob had won thirteen races including several valuable prizes. "His choice, by a panel of more than twenty journalists and television commentators, was entirely on merit," John Watt confirmed. "He was quite simply the most successful jockey of the month and it was an unprecedented feat to win such a coveted award twice in three months. It had never happened before in any of the racing awards we run." The *Guardian* carried a lengthy story about Bob's award under a headline FIVE STAR CHAMPION.

Bob received his inscribed whip and a cheque for a hundred gallons of petrol at a reception laid on by the Amoco sponsors at the Cheltenham festival meeting in mid-March. An important absentee from Cheltenham was Aldaniti, who had done so well since his victory at Ascot in February that Josh Gifford was greatly tempted to let him run in the Tote Cheltenham Gold Cup on the Thursday. The race, Josh reasoned, was wide open and the horse had an obvious chance. But after considerable discussion the horse's owner Nick Embiricos decided, much to Bob's relief, that the horse would miss Cheltenhan and not run before the Grand National. Nick Embiricos pointed out that Aldaniti had already finished third in the Gold Cup, was unlikely to improve on that performance and the testing going after heavy rain would inevitably put a severe strain on his suspect front legs. Bob rode Approaching in the Gold Cup. They moved into fourth place briefly a mile from home but faded in the closing stages.

Chapter 17

THE 1981 GRAND National meeting could not have started more disastrously for Josh Gifford, Nick and Valda Embiricos and all those who supported the impossible dream that Aldaniti and Bob Champion would win the Grand National on the Saturday. Valda Embiricos was quite hopeful that her honest and consistent horse Stonepark, trained by Josh, had a fine chance in the Topham Trophy on Thursday, the first race of the meeting over the Grand National fences. Stonepark, aged nine, had won six races despite missing the previous season with leg trouble. Back in form, ridden at ten stone by Richard Rowe, he started one of the favourites in a field of eighteen.

The first fence in the Topham Trophy is the twenty-ninth in the Grand National, a relatively small jump at Liverpool, 4 feet 7 inches high with the usual covering of fir and spruce. Stonepark took off well enough but overjumped, landed on his nose and fell heavily. At first he seemed all right but as he struggled to his feet and tried to gallop off racegoers on the grandstand and viewers watching on television realized in horror that he was seriously injured. Clearly in pain he attempted to continue in the race riderless. Finally he was caught and after an uncomfortably long delay a vet diagnosed that he had broken his neck in the fall. There was only one option. Stonepark was destroyed.

Poor Valda Embiricos was overcome with grief. Her husband, too, was deeply upset. The couple were so distressed at the death of Stonepark that for a few minutes Nick decided to withdraw Aldaniti from the Grand National to avoid the possibility of further anguish on Saturday. It was but a momentary hesitation and happily Nick Embiricos quickly reconsidered his verdict. Aldaniti was already on his way to Liverpool. After so much patience and planning Nick decided it was too late for an eleventh hour change of mind. "Until it happened I had forgotten how cruel this course could be. Just for a moment I thought I couldn't let Aldaniti run. But so much was involved for so many people that my courage came back."

But the drama of the day was not over. In the last race of the afternoon Bob rode Kilbroney who was making a steady comeback after a leg injury. Kilbroney was well enough placed when he completely misjudged the eighth fence, the water jump, directly in front of the stands. He took off much too far away, landed in the water and when his hind legs slipped under him, his jockey, with nothing to sit on, rolled heavily face down onto the ground. As Bob lay still Sunrise Hill, a backmarker, appeared to kick him on his back and head. His body jerked like a rag doll and he rolled in agony for a few seconds.

For one moment I thought my chance of riding in the National had gone. Luckily his hoof missed my head but he still kicked me in the middle of the back and for just an instant I feared I'd had it. It was more painful than anything else.

White-faced, clearly distressed, Bob dragged himself on to his knees, eventually stood up, back bent and shoulders hunched, and limped off to the safety of the rails before making his way slowly towards the jockeys' changing-room where he told the doctor that he was unharmed. When he peeled off his colours he discovered a vivid scarlet imprint of Sunrise Hill's hoof on his back.

It could have been a lot worse. I'm glad to get a fall out of the way before the National. I've not had one for weeks. After a sauna and a hot bath I'll be all right.

Southport's sauna, close to the sea front, has long been a refuge for Grand National jockeys. There on Thursday evening Bob was able to relax for an hour or two before joining Jo for dinner at a nearby Italian restaurant with the Embiricos family, Josh and Althea Gifford, Henry Pelham and several other friends including Monty Court, John Oaksey, and—a latecomer, as usual—Brough Scott. While the rest of us worked our way through an excellent menu Bob restricted himself to a lone piece of fish without any vegetables and sipped a glass of wine.

The morning before the National he left the hotel at seven o'clock to ride Aldaniti in a short canter on the racecourse. He returned two hours later declaring jubilantly,

> The horse is spot on. I've never known him better. He's travelled up well and eaten everything he's been given. Even though we cantered for only three furlongs, twice, he was eager and took a right hold.

After breakfast Bob returned to the sauna with Bill Smith and Philip Blacker, who were also riding in the Grand National. Philip, a gifted sculptor, had already been approached by Nick and Valda Embiricos to do a bronze of Aldaniti. Bill had come in for the ride on Coolishall after Brod Munro-Wilson, the horse's owner, trainer and amateur rider had dislocated his shoulder and broken some ribs in a fall at Liverpool on Thursday. The morning sauna helped ease Bob's back which had stiffened overnight and though he felt some discomfort after finishing unplaced in a novice hurdle, his only ride of the day, he reported that the injury had not been a problem.

> At least I'm in one piece to ride in the National now. I've made it even if I make a fool of myself and fall off at the first fence.

The previous weekend Bob had given an intriguing insight in the *Sunday People* into his chances in the race. Under an ambitious two-page headline, I'LL WIN IT FOR YOU ALL he explained that the first two fences might be a problem.

> Aldaniti is such a bold, at times extravagant, jumper I'm worried he might overjump. But he should adapt quickly enough. I'll be happy if I can get him to relax for the first 3½ miles. He can run away after that. If everything goes right and we have a clear round, then whatever finishes in front of us will win.
>
> Spartan Missile and Royal Mail are the only other class horses in the race. Don't be put off by Spartan Missile's jockey John Thorne. who is old enough to be my father and will probably

carry a few pounds overweight. I was very impressed with both of them when they finished fourth in the Gold Cup at Cheltenham. No man could have given the horse a better ride.

Two other National runners that interest me are the 1979 winner Rubstic and Martinstown. When I worked for Toby Balding I broke in Rubstic as a yearling and rode him every day; I even schooled him over hurdles as a two-year-old. He was a very good jumper but seemed the slowest thing I'd ever sat on. I rode one of my first winners on Martinstown's mother Last Town way back in 1968. Last Town was a fine tough old mare and her son has clearly inherited some of her best qualities, but basically Aldaniti has much more class than Rubstic, Martinstown and most of the field.

I badly want to win the race for so many people, in particular the doctors and nurses who kept me going when all hope seemed gone. I also want to win for Josh who kept my job waiting for me and then helped me through a bad patch when the horses were wrong and my confidence was rock bottom. Few, if any, trainers would have done the same. My family, friends and many owners were terrific too. Nick and Valda Embiricos sent me get well cards and I even had one from Aldaniti who has his own fan club organized by their daughter Alexandra.

But most of all I want to win the Grand National for all the patients still in hospital. If any success I have can give people fresh heart and just a bit of hope then everything that has happened to me in the past twenty months will have been worthwhile.

After racing on Friday Bob had time for another hour in the Southport sauna, though he was very happy about his weight in the National.

My weight was really quite good. Aldaniti was set to carry 10 stone 13 pounds in the race. If Josh and I had written to the handicapper pleading for leniency we couldn't have expected a better weight. Aldaniti was one of the only three class horses in the race yet was incredibly well handicapped. That enabled me to ride on my middle saddle, my favourite one, which weighs about three pounds. That might sound very light when you consider the average saddle used for hunting or riding weighs around a stone or even more. But small saddles have become part of my life. My lightest is two pounds. That's quite heavy by the standards of some flat race jockeys. Lester Piggott's lightest saddle, for instance, fully equipped, is just a fraction under a pound.

Early that evening everyone crowded into Nick and Valda Embiricos's bedroom to watch Bob's interview on *Nationwide*, the first of several television appearances in the next twenty-four hours. Nick and Valda's four children—Nicholas, Alastair, Euan and Alexandra—had travelled up to support Aldaniti and the party also included Josh and Althea Gifford's Border terrier Rocky. After *Nationwide* came Bob's guest appearance on *A Question of Sport*. He answered his questions well but his team, captained by Emlyn Hughes, lost narrowly on the last point of the quiz.

Dinner on Friday night gradually developed into a pre-race celebration. As the evening wore on defeat for Aldaniti the following afternoon seemed an increasingly remote possibility. Bob limited himself to a small helping of chicken and declined all offers of alcohol. Soon after eleven o'clock, when the party had all drifted back to the hotel, he announced that he was going to bed. Josh Gifford, who had known several Grand National winning jockeys behave riotously the night before the race, took him to one side and told him to go off to a club and have a few drinks if he wanted to and not to bother about having an early night. Bob, who was certainly the most relaxed man in the group, declined such well intentioned advice and set off up the stairs with Jo to raucous applause. Whatever anyone else thought or said he did not intend to throw away his chance the next day through extravagant behaviour in the clubs of Southport in the early hours of the morning.

We are all different. I've known some jockeys go out on the town all night, finish up legless, yet ride brilliant races the next day. I am not like that. I'm not a drinker and particularly since my weight has been so bad I've had to watch myself all the time. Some of the boys think that drinking heavily the night before the National helps them sleep when they finally get to bed. Well, believe it or not, I was still calm and I slept soundly.

Dawn on Saturday 4th April promised a golden sunny day. As we drove to the course at seven a.m. Bob laughed, "I hope it stays like this all day. I always ride much better with the sun on my back." He cantered both Aldaniti and Homeson, who he was riding later in the day, then set off to walk the course with Nick and Valda Embiricos and their four children, Henry Pelham, Josh and Althea Gifford, their son Nick and, inevitably, Rocky, the terrier. Three days of sunshine had dried the ground considerably but Liverpool, like most of the country, had suffered the wettest March for many years and the going in places was still surprisingly testing. Footholes, some twelve inches or more deep, remained from the two races over the National course on Thursday.

The Grand National is one of the finest, most dramatic sporting spectacles of our age, the ultimate test of horse and rider, an incomparable event of consuming intensity. Millions who care little for horses and even less for betting continue to be enthralled by the sight of colourful fields of steeplechasers tackling the awesome, unique fences, big solid obstacles consisting of thick birch stakes, growing four feet or more above the ground, lavishly covered with spruce and fir. Walking the National course is a chastening experience for newcomers and experienced racegoers alike. After a year spent racing at courses with smaller, narrower and much easier fences, the massive green jumps of Liverpool seemed impossibly large. The first fence is not particularly big, just 4 feet 6 inches high, but the unusually long run from the start, the large number of runners and the inevitable tension invariably combine to cause a few fallers there. In 1951 eleven of the thirty-six starters fell at the first fence, and Bob's National hopes had twice ended there. On Saturday morning he studied it for a moment, then smiled.

Once you are here it's too late to change your mind. One of the chief problems is that horse and rider can't see over any of the fences so there is always the danger of being brought down by a loose horse or faller, something that happened to me on my first ride in the race. So you just pray you have a clear landing and don't overjump.

The second fence, just an inch higher than the first, does not normally cause problems, but the third is the most feared hazard in the early part of the race: five feet high, unusually wide, with a six-feet ditch in front of it, it provides a severe test to horses used to jumping more conventional ditches elsewhere. Bob confessed he was worried about this fence.

> It catches a lot of horses out. Once we are over it safely we can start to think about riding a race. You can see why soft or duck-hearted horses don't like the course. The ones that frighten themselves don't last much longer than the third.

After examining the first three fences Josh decided that Bob should start the race on the wide outside on Aldaniti. The drops on the landing side, he reasoned, were less severe there and the ground was marginally better. The fourth and fifth fences are relatively straightforward for horses that have survived the early cavalry charge but number six, Becher's Brook, is the most famous fence on the course, marked by a huge fluttering flag bearing a white 'B'. It is named after Captain Becher who fell there on Conrad in 1839, the first year of the race, and wisely threw himself into the ditch to avoid the thundering hooves of the opposition until remounting once they had passed. Anyone walking round the course would be surprised at the smallness of the fence on the take-off side since it is just 4 feet 10 inches high. A tiny brook runs along the bottom of the landing side where all the considerable trouble is caused by the sudden and unexpectedly deep drop, particularly on the inside. Many horses are unable to cope with this severe slope; some take off too soon and pitch too steeply on landing. Others take off too close, hit the fence hard and tip over.

Bob and Josh moved on to the next fence, the seventh on the first circuit and twenty-third on the second. It is one of the smallest and most innocuous obstacles on the course but sometimes causes problems because it is so different from the previous jump. It is the fence that Josh Gifford remembers most from his many attempts at the Grand National because, he firmly believes, it cost him victory in 1967.

Josh finished second on Honey End, the favourite that year when Foinavon, a 100-1 outsider, was the only horse to avoid an unprecedented pile-up caused by two loose horses at the fence on the second circuit. The race leaders found their paths blocked and stopped abruptly, dislodging their jockeys; other runners close behind were baulked and the rest of the field was halted by a traffic jam of rush-hour proportions. Some horses struggled across the fence without their jockeys. Some jockeys were sent tumbling over the remains of the fence without their mounts, then scrambled despairingly around the birch in an equine parody of musical chairs. In a moment of panic at least one jockey remounted the wrong horse. Foinavon and his young jockey John Buckingham were the only pair to avoid the mêlée. Jinking their way through the chaos with nimble skill they arrived at the shattered fence at little more than a trot, popped safely over and galloped off in splendid isolation. Josh Gifford was stopped twice on Honey End by other horses before he was able to set off in distant pursuit but by then Foinavon had stolen an unassailable lead. Honey End, despite making up an enormous amount of ground finished second, beaten by fifteen lengths. "Yes," says Josh, "I think I would have won all right if there hadn't been a pile-up—but so do six other jockeys who were still going well!"

Fence number eight on the Grand National Course is the Canal Turn, perhaps the most spectacular of all. The course turns left-handed at ninety degrees immediately after the jump and the cleverest horses cross it at an angle to save precious ground on landing. The Canal Turn is big—five feet high—and was the scene of another famous mêlée in 1928 when Easter Hero straddled it on the first circuit and caused so much confusion that he put most of the field out of the race. The original Canal Turn was a monster by modern standards, but later it was modified and protected by railings in a bid to stop runners galloping headlong into the old Leeds–Liverpool waterway.

As they walked round, Bob and Josh discovered that the ground on the inside of the course near the Canal Turn was soft and badly chewed up after the two races on Thursday. That strengthened their resolve that Aldaniti should keep to the better going on the wide outside on the first circuit at least. The four fences after the Canal Turn include three more ditches. Valentine's Brook, number nine, is more than five feet high with a brook 5 feet 6 inches wide on the landing side.

It's a lovely fence for a good bold jumper. Mind you, I fell there on Shifting Gold in 1978. He was a good jumper elsewhere but a bit small for Liverpool and had shown no sign of adapting at all from the start. He made several bad mistakes and it was just a matter of time before we hit the ground.

A plain fence is followed by two more ditches—at the eleventh on the take-off side of the fence and at the twelfth on the landing side—before a long, sweeping left-handed run leads towards the next two jumps, both plain and slightly smaller. These are the final two fences of the race on the second circuit but on the first lap two more remain, including the water jump and the massive Chair—the most frightening obstacle of all. The Chair is 5 feet 2 inches high and is guarded by a huge, gaping ditch, six feet wide on the take-off side. It is a spectacular, formidable and unique landmark in front of the stands and some horses are simply not able to leap high enough and far enough to cross it safely.

Half the problem is that it's so narrow that you can't expect too much daylight. If you are behind you don't know what's happening on the landing side. It's the fence that sorts out the men from the boys. If I can be handy here on Aldaniti at the end of the first circuit I'll be happy.

After walking a complete circuit of two and a quarter miles the party paused by the Chair fence before heading back to the car park. Nick Embiricos said quietly, "The most important thing is that horse and jockey are here in one piece. Whatever happens this afternoon that is a major achievement."

Several experts in the morning papers tipped Aldaniti to win but even that combined display of confidence did not worry the horse's jockey.

I felt unusually relaxed. When I came back to the hotel from the sauna just before midday. I had a glass of champagne with Josh and the owners who were all wound up. They seemed a bit worried that I was too calm.

In the car on the way back to the racecourse Jo suggested that Bob had fulfilled his long-held obsession to regain his fitness to ride Aldaniti in the Grand National and perhaps that was all that mattered. Bob's reaction was emphatic.

You must be joking! Now I've come this far I intend to bloody well win the race, and I've got the toughest possible horse going into battle with me.

Numerous good luck messages and telegrams awaited him at the weighing-room. Sally and Nigel Dimmer from Cheltenham sent a massive card and a minute silver horseshoe with instructions that it should be carried by him in the race. A card from his parents read simply, "May you be first past the post." There was a telegram from his sister Mary, her husband Richard and their two children Emma and Nicky. Another telegram said simply, "Be lucky from Jude and all at Findon." Bob's cousins Sarah and Julie sent a card enclosing two coloured pills which looked suspiciously like Smarties and guaranteed a hundred per cent success rate; the black one to be taken fifteen minutes before the race and the green one at the command for jockeys to mount their horses in the paddock.

There were many more from people he did not know. An old age pensioner wrote: "Having read you in the *Sunday People* my prayers, your hopes and my wager will be on you on Saturday, and if you are 'pipped' (perhaps by John Thorne) I know you will accept it like the sportsman and gentleman you are. Above all please, please be careful."

Another letter began, "What a great name you have to match the great guy you are. In the *People* you made me and, I'm sure, millions of others feel very ashamed of grumbling at our pains and moans. I do hope you'll forgive me for writing but I'd like you to know, as you ride, that I'll be jumping up and down like a maniac to will you and Aldaniti on."

Audrey and Chas Castle from Crowhurst sent a good luck card saying, "May you have wings to take you up and over all thirty fences and some puff at the end. Happy landings."

A nurse who had worked in the hospital where he had been treated wrote: "I remember working in the Pinkham ward and nursing you. My memories of you are not exactly happy ones as you were undergoing chemotherapy and in the depths of despair. But just before I left the hospital I remember you stopping me excitedly just outside the outpatients' department where you told me the doctors had given you the fantastic news that your treatment had been a success and you were all clear. I can still remember your face as I had never seen you smile before in several months. I wish you luck in the Grand National and I shall have a few bob riding on you."

Bob was overwhelmed.

I've never had so much post in all my life, and most of it was from people I hadn't even met. It was just like having Christmas and my birthday at the same time. I was very touched that everyone had taken the trouble to write to me.

Bob's ride on Aldaniti in the Grand National, due to start at 3.20, was his first of the afternoon. Before the first race he was whisked by a fast car the few furlongs to Becher's Brook and stood in the deepest part of the drop on the landing side of the fence for an interview with David Coleman as part of the build-up for the BBC television's *Grandstand* programme. He returned to the winning post just in time to see the opening Sunratings Chase and then he walked to the weighing-room to change into the distinctive colours of Nick Embiricos that he would wear on Aldaniti—a white rollneck jersey with a royal blue sash, armlets and cap. "At least you'll be able to spot me when I fall off," he told one amused commentator.

As he busied himself in the changing-room, checking his boots and breeches and the stirrup leathers on his saddle, the tension of the day at last began to affect him.

I was still reasonably relaxed. The trouble is that you have to get to the course so early to avoid the possibility of being held up in the traffic and then you are left to wander around the racecourse with hours to kill before the race. As long as I'm doing something I'm fine but I hate waiting around. I sat on the practice scales a couple of times, looked at a few newspapers, watched a race at Salisbury on television and wandered around chatting to some of the boys riding in the race. I also popped out to see Carol and Jenny who I had invited to come up by train for the day from London. I had arranged grandstand tickets for the girls and I made sure they were all right. It was strange seeing them both at a racecourse on such an important day because there were so many times in hospital when they and I must have felt my chances of riding in a race, let alone the National, were a million to one.

Bob watched the second race on television in the jockeys' room, then weighed out and found that he could manage the correct mark of 10 stone 13 comfortably. The combined weight of the saddle, a foam pad to go underneath it, and a breastplate to prevent the saddle slipping back amounted to almost five pounds. Bob waited impassively as the clerk of the scales checked his weight then passed the tack to 68-year-old Snowy Davis, a marvellous character with a wrinkled leathery face, who had worked in racing since 1926 and had been travelling head lad for Josh Gifford since he started training. Then there was yet more time to waste.

The next twenty minutes or so are the worst of all. Most of the jockeys have passed the scales. A few more are still waiting to do so. Some sit down quietly. Others, like me, pace endlessly. You begin to wonder what the hell you are doing riding in such a race and wish you were hundreds of miles away in London having a few drinks while watching the Boat Race. Anywhere but Liverpool.

You are about to tackle the biggest fences in the business and the whole world is waiting to see you make a fool of yourself. Somehow the time passes but so slowly. Each minute seems to last an hour. I had a few sips from a bottle of Lucozade I'd brought with me and watched more races on television from Salisbury and Stockton and some of the interviews David Coleman held with jockeys riding in the National. There was a constant stream of jockeys going to the gents. I put the silver horseshoe that had been sent to me in one of my boots, added a sprig of heather I'd been given for good luck and washed off my goggles. For the first time I can remember, one of the stewards didn't come in and warn us about the dangers of going too fast too early. I never understood why he bothered anyway. Everyone used to burst out laughing as soon as he'd gone. Not that he was particularly funny. It was just a way of relieving the tension.

Finally it's time to go. We wish each other luck and file out past the waiting television camera trained on the door of the weighing-room.

The paddock at Aintree is barely able to cope with thirty-nine horses plus the usual gaggle of jockeys, owners, trainers, lads and officials. The horses were led round in two circles. Bob, showing no sign of the growing tension, walked briskly into the parade ring, moved across to join Aldaniti's party, touched his cap and folded his arms as he chatted quietly with Josh Gifford.

"Well, we've got this far," said Josh. "You know what to do and the best of luck." Bob explains.

There was no need for orders. We'd been through the race a dozen times in the previous weeks. Josh and I both felt Aldaniti, Spartan Missile and Royal Mail were the only class horses of the race. Our plan was to try to keep out of trouble on the first circuit and then think about winning.

When I'd just been beaten on Aldaniti in the Scottish Grand National in 1979 I came back convinced I would have won if I had taken the lead much earlier—as much as a mile and a half from home. This time Josh and I were sure Aldaniti would stay but we hoped I'd have a nice lead for most of the way. As the horses walked round the paddock I thought Aldaniti looked superb. He's a lovely old-fashioned stamp of steeplechaser and was in tremendous condition.

Josh Gifford legged Bob into the saddle and the horse's lad, nineteen-year-old Peter Double led them round the paddock once before they set off for the long parade in front of the stands. The thirty-nine runners walked down the course on the hurdle track in front of the stands towards the Chair fence and then turned to canter back past the starting point towards the first fence.

The horse was calm throughout and I was not at all nervous once I was in the paddock. It was just another race, another job to do.

I'm getting a bit too old for pre-race nerves. Aldaniti was in great form and took a strong hold cantering down. He was very free. We had a look at the first fence then cantered back to the start where Josh was waiting to help tighten the girths on my saddle.

Nick Henderson, the young trainer of Zongalero, second in the race in 1979, was also at the start to check his horse's girths. Nick said he had given up smoking and Josh immediately agreed to do the same if Aldaniti won—a rash promise since he was a heavy smoker.

The huge field of runners circling colourfully at the start in bright sunshine contained several horses and jockeys whose chances of finishing, let alone winning, were remote. On the morning of the race six horses were on offer at 100-1, four more were freely available at 200-1 while two were dismissed at 500-1. One of this pair, Deiopea, was ridden by housewife Linda Sheedy, aged 28, hoping to become the first woman rider to finish in the Grand National. A mother of nine-year-old twin boys, Linda, a small chatty blonde, both feminine and tough, was not at all deterred by the fact that she had already suffered a series of appalling injuries in race falls, including a shattered right leg and ankle held together by three pins, two screws and a plate.

Moving beside Deiopea was Dromore, ridden by his enthusiastic owner-trainer Peter Duggan, an Irishman who spent six months of each year working on an oil rig in the North Sea. Another forlorn outsider was Bryan Boru, ridden by a 44-year-old Cheshire solicitor, John Carden, at considerable overweight. Carden had crashed several times at Aintree in his days as a motor-racing driver and his fortune at the course had not improved when he switched to steeplechasing. He had ended up in hospital after four of his five previous attempts over the Grand National fences and Bryan Boru's dismal form offered little prospect of a painless conclusion to his venture this time.

The tallest jockey in the race, his sole earring glinting in the sun, was a 6 feet 3 inches amateur rider, Malcolm Batters, on Martinstown, owned and trained by Bob's old friend Mrs Mita Easton. Malcolm Batters was the barman at her pub the Sheaf of Arrows. An even more unlikely amateur rider was the eccentric Aidan O'Connell on Chumson. Built like a rugby forward, 6 feet 2 inches tall, Aidan O'Connell was that rare animal, an Irish dandy. In the final weeks before the 1981 Grand National, Aidan's occasional presence in the Hungerford sauna had helped make Bob's constant battle with the scales more bearable. Bob even offered Aidan 10-1 against finishing in front of him.

Three days after Aidan broke his shoulder at the first fence in the 1979 Grand National he was hiking along a lonely Berkshire lane to his temporary stables a few miles away. Eventually he was given a lift by an ancient yokel in an even more ancient, battered car. Aidan, dressed flamboyantly as usual, folded his huge frame into the back seat of the car while nursing his shoulder in a sling. Progress along the road was not exactly spectacular. After five minutes and perhaps twenty yards the driver asked, "How did you hurt yourself?"

"I had a kick," said Aidan.

"That's a funny place to have a kick."

"Ah, I was on the ground at the time," he replied.

"What were you doing there?"

"I'd had a fall."

"A fall," mused the driver.

"Yes, from a racehorse," answered Aidan.

By now the car had covered at least one hundred yards but the driver was eyeing his passenger through the mirror with increasing suspicion.

"You were riding in a race?" he asked incredulously.

"Yes, at Liverpool."

"Never," hissed the driver.

"Yes, as a matter of fact it was in last Saturday's Grand National," said Aidan. The car slowed to a halt, the driver leaped out, walked round to the rear door and held it open.

"Get out of my car!" he cried. "I won't have any more of your lies. You can walk the rest of the way."

Thus Aidan O'Connell, for the first time in his life, was rendered speechless.

But the most astonishing rider in the 1981 race was surely grandfather John Thorne, owner, breeder, trainer and jockey of the massive steeplechaser Spartan Missile, the long-time favourite for the race. Spartan Missile was an entirely worthy favourite. Twice winner of the Foxhunters Chase over the Grand National fences, he jumped well, possessed unlimited stamina and seemed an ideal National prospect.

John Thorne, a farmer and Master of Foxhounds might reasonably be expected to have given up the role of jockey at the advanced age of 54, especially as his weight had long before settled agreeably at a conservative figure of 13½ stone. Giving up, however, had never been easy for a man like Thorne and two experiences in his life had made it a particularly difficult thing for him to do. One was that aged just seventeen crossing the Rhine with the Sixth Airborne Division towards the end of the war and landing in a glider seven miles behind the German lines must have made the considerable hazards of steeplechasing seem almost harmless in comparison. The other was the tragic death of his son Nigel in December 1968, just as he was establishing himself as a dashing young jockey. As a result his father postponed his retirement from the saddle indefinitely.

John Thorne once broke his back so badly in a race fall that doctors warned him he should not ride again. Treating that well intentioned advice with an ill-concealed disdain that Bob Champion could not have bettered, John spent several painful months recovering, resumed racing and in 1966 won the National Hunt Chase at Cheltenham on Polaris Missile, the dam of Spartan Missile. In the 1981 Grand National Spartan Missile was set to carry 11 stone 2 pounds, a weight which launched John Thorne on a self denial programme of such brutal proportions that he lived on a diet of fresh air and grapefruit in the weeks before the race and shed over two stone. On the day he carried just three pounds overweight at 11 stone 5, his lightest for twenty years.

Chapter 18

DURING THE FINAL hectic seconds of betting before the race began, Spartan Missile was backed down to 8-1 with Aldaniti second favourite at 10-1 and the 1979 winner Rubstic at 11-1. Nick Embiricos was unimpressed by such odds. Back in December he had asked Josh Gifford to place a bet of five hundred pounds each way at 66-1 on Aldaniti. Josh—who was entitled to adopt a more cautious approach so long before Liverpool—instead invested £250 each way.

A few moments after 3.20 the thirty-nine runners, ready to compete for a first prize of £51,324, moved up to the starting tapes and began to sort themselves into a semblance of order. Some jockeys, like the brilliant double champion John Francome on So and Philip Blacker on the top weight Royal Mail, opted for the inside where the advantage of fewer horses was offset perhaps by the steeper drops they would encounter. A dozen horses and riders joined Bob Champion on the wide outside of the course. Bob walked round quietly on Aldaniti watching carefully as the starter, Captain Dick Smalley, mounted his rostrum. A white flag was raised and a few seconds later, to an expectant roar, Captain Smalley pressed the lever in his hand, the tapes rose and the field for the 1981 Grand National surged off towards the first fence some four hundred and fifty yards away. Bob Champion's distinctive white colours could be seen on Aldaniti on the outside.

I had an ideal position. I didn't want to be in the front rank. My plan was to settle Aldaniti a bit so I walked him out of the gate in the second row and he was running away at once. When you walk round it seems a hell of a long run to the first but it doesn't take many seconds in a race. Halfway there you cross the Melling Road covered especially for the day. Fred Winter, who won the race twice as a jockey, had advised me to take a pull and get him back on his hocks immediately after crossing that road. I managed to do that though we all seemed to be going a right gallop.

As we came to the fence Aldaniti stood off far too far away, pinged it, but came down much too steep. I slipped my reins to the end of the buckle but I thought we had gone. What a waste for both of us. He was on the ground, down. His nose and knees scraping the grass. We'd had it. Yet somehow he came back up and we were still in one piece. A lot of horses would have gone over in that position. He was much too eager just as we had feared. He found a leg, regained his balance and I hoped it had taught him a valuable lesson.

But the second fence wasn't much better. When he reached it he stood off even further and almost landed on top of it though he never felt like falling. He scraped his belly on it. That hurt him and taught him an even sharper lesson.

There wasn't time to worry. Either he'd adapt soon or we'd be parting company. The big ditch, the third, surprised him, almost frightened him a little. But he's as brave as a lion and didn't flinch. He's the sort of horse that gives you everything he's got. Going to the fourth I had to give him a kick in the belly to organize him to take off and from then on he realized what he had to do. He's a very intelligent horse and those early fences made him think. Even though he was running quite free he was having a look at them. After the first three fences he was quite brilliant. I just sat on him after that. A complete passenger. You see, the fences are so big and wide a horse has to be sensible and adapt or fall. If you try to take every fence on you are bound to end up on the floor. Aldaniti, who had never fallen in his life, quickly learned to get in a bit closer to the fences and pop over them. Although he was pulling hard he knew what to do each time we reached a fence.

There seemed to be a wall of horses in front of us at Becher's and if anything had fallen there I'd have been in trouble. He jumped it well, towards the rear, just behind The Vintner who is not the safest of jumpers so I thought I'd better move past him.

Approaching the eighth fence, the Canal Turn, six horses, including Bryan Boru, were already out of the race. Carrow Boy led there from Choral Festival, Tenecoon and Zongalero. Aldaniti, in twentieth position, gained several lengths as he soared gloriously over it. Three fences later his gallant white face was showing in front. There it remained as a series of quite breathtaking matchless leaps steadily took him clear of the others. Bob Champion was as surprised as anyone by his sudden surge to the front.

I thought, What the hell am I doing here? Aldaniti was enjoying himself and was gaining two or three lengths at each fence. He was measuring them perfectly and was so quick at getting away from them on landing.

I didn't want to be in front so soon and I was sure Josh didn't want me there either. But I had no choice. Aldaniti had taken me there. It was just like Snow Flyer at Newbury. I got a bollocking there and it was going through my mind that if I got beaten now I was sure to get another one; and it would be deserved. I was there far too soon. I'd have been mad with myself if I'd been beaten. I didn't go there on purpose. I got there without trying. Josh knew he was difficult to ride so I hoped he would understand.

The trouble was that Aldaniti was still so keen to get on with it. It didn't worry me that my strength would run out. I was sure I was stronger and fitter than before my illness. The way I felt at that moment I could have held a moving mountain all day, but it was a problem that he was doing too much all the time, especially as his legs were not the best in the world. Usually I was able to get him switched off in a race by sticking him right up another horse's backside, then he wouldn't pull at all. I'd been hoping to have a lead to the last fence.

But it was too late for that. His superior class and jumping ability had carried him to the front sooner than anyone would have wanted. There was no point in hauling him back. I just hoped he would settle better in front.

Far from settling, Aldaniti could be seen shaking his head from side to side, pulling his jockey's arms out, as he led the field back across the Melling Road towards the grandstand. Skipping gaily over the 'hirteenth and fourteenth fences Aldaniti headed for the dreaded

Chair with Zongalero, Royal Stuart and Rubstic in close attendance and Spartan Missile and Royal Mail handily placed.

Aldaniti made nothing of the Chair. He saw a nice long stride, stood off and really pinged it. He must have been good because all the photographs show me sitting up his neck like a flat jockey and you don't see that very often. He popped over the water and going out on the second circuit I tried to find the ridge of good ground in the middle of the course. Aldaniti was still running away at that stage. Rubstic was on my inside and Royal Stuart on my outside and neither of them seemed to be going as well.

I was still a bit unhappy about being in front for so long but I began to think I might have a chance of winning if I kept my head. I kept telling myself to think like a jockey and not get too excited. Going to the first fence on the second circuit, the seventeenth, we were upsides with Rubstic yet we landed four lengths clear. My horse was absolutely brilliant. Royal Stuart joined us at the next but once again my fellow must have gained three or four lengths because I never saw Royal Stuart again. Aldaniti was so quick away from his fences. I'd ridden at Liverpool in one race or another many times but I'd never sat on anything that jumped there like Aldaniti. He was like a cat, so fast, so sure and loving every minute of it. He's my type of horse. So genuine and honest. He would never shirk from anything.

But a jockey can get so wrapped up with the excitement of jumping that he forgets about riding a race. The further we went the more I realized we might win if I didn't do anything silly. By the time we got to Becher's we were a few lengths clear. I pulled him out a bit so I could jump it on the angle nearer the inside, so I could save a bit of ground which I did.

Aldaniti soared breathtakingly over the fence, pitched on landing and was picked up effortlessly by his jockey as Pacify fell behind him in second place. After the next two—Rubstic and Royal Mail—there was a gap of a dozen lengths or more to the following group which included Senator Maclacury, Three to One, Royal Exile, and Spartan Missile who had lost his good position after a mistake early on the second circuit.

Ivor Markham, a former jockey and experienced race reader, was standing on the landing side of Becher's Brook. He reports: "Aldaniti jumped it well, almost too well and peckèd really badly as he landed. His nose hit the ground and the pictures of the incident show just how perilous his position was. Yet Bob is such a fine horseman that he picked him smoothly up and made it seem as though nothing had happened." According to Bob, nothing much *had* happened.

He nodded there all right but always felt safe. Basically if they don't nod at Becher's they don't have a chance of standing up. By now I was thinking if I use my brains I'll win this. We popped over the twenty-third and at the next, the Canal Turn, I aimed him in at an angle, asked him to stand off and he was out of this world. What a horse! I stood him off the next one too. He was still going like a dream, strong and powerful and jumping from fence to fence. I kept trying to give him little breathers between the fences, to get a bit of oxygen into his lungs. His legs felt fine, he hadn't faltered at all.

Heading towards the third last fence Rubstic fell away beaten leaving Aldaniti tracked by Royal Mail with a gap back to Three to One, Senator Maclacury and Spartan Missile who was at last starting to make up the lost ground. Bob was out on his own.

I knew my fellow would keep galloping. There had never been any doubts about his stamina and he was far too brave to give in. He came to third last slightly wrong so I let him drift into the corner and he just flicked the top without harm. Then I heard another horse immediately behind us.

It was Royal Mail whose jockey Philip Blacker was still confident of victory: "My horse was doing it well and economically and giving me the best ride I've ever had at Liverpool. I always hoped I would catch Aldaniti. But all the time I thought Bob's horse was doing it a little bit easier. He was floating."

Aldaniti headed back across the Melling Road, two lengths clear of Royal Mail. Ten lengths or so behind came Three to One and

Senator Maclacury just ahead of Spartan Missile who was still making steady progress. By now the thousands at Aintree and millions watching on television began to realize they were witnessing the moving climax to surely the most unlikely and emotional comeback in the history of sport. Bob Champion, so gravely ill eighteen months earlier, and Aldaniti, whose career had been beset by injuries, had been in front for more than a circuit and were still going strongly. But would the horse have the endurance to last the final torturous stretch after such a light preparation, and would his jockey have the necessary strength and fitness to help him do so?

I didn't feel at all tired—I was too busy concentrating! Every time I thought I might win I kept telling myself not to be stupid. The long run to the second last seemed to go on for ever. I was sure of Aldaniti's stamina so I gave him a slap down the shoulder and tried to keep increasing and increasing the pace. I knew someone was close behind and had a couple of peeps to see how he was going. On the final bend I deliberately kept wide, as Josh and I had planned, to find the better going. Approaching the second last Aldaniti was beginning to feel a bit tired and his old tongue came lolling out on the right hand side, which was a sure sign that he was tired. But I knew he would keep going. I headed back for the tight inside of the second last, Aldaniti jumped it well, and I wasn't sorry to hear a crash immediately behind me as something made a bad mistake. Now I was thinking: There's only one more fence to jump and we must be in with a chance.

My horse takes a lot of riding and holding together and it was obvious he was weary. The finish still seemed miles away. I realized he was meeting the last fence wrong but I had no intention of asking him to take off too far away and risking putting him on the ground. That would have been madness. He was much too tired for that. So I allowed him to run into the corner and pop over to be safe, then once we had landed I pulled my stick through into my right hand and gave him a slap down the shoulder and a crack round the backside just to remind him he still had some work to do.

I could see another horse out of the corner of my eye—it got to within perhaps a length of us—then Aldaniti rolled a bit left-handed as though he thought he had to jump the Chair fence again since, for the first half of that long, endless run-in, there is no running rail to help horses. He was giving everything he had to offer but he was desperately tired, so I just tried to concentrate on holding him together and keeping him balanced.

I've always thought I'm a better jockey in front than behind. I'm a good judge of pace and I love riding from the front but this time I wished I could see behind me to find out if anything was finishing strongly. That run-in at Liverpool can be the loneliest place in the world. I was only too aware that in the past several horses had been caught and passed there after leading for a long way.

Some way behind, Spartan Missile was making up ground at an astonishing rate at the end of such a gruelling race. He had jumped into third place at the final fence, ten lengths behind Aldaniti, and set off in pursuit as if he had just joined the race as a fresh horse. Certainly during the first half of the run-in his relentless gallop took him closer to Aldaniti with every stride, and for a few, tense, critical moments it seemed Bob Champion and his valiant partner might suffer the heartbreak of being caught in the last despairing yards of an epic race.

When we got to the elbow, halfway up the run-in, Aldaniti had a rail to help him. He was so tired by then but he still had the strength to keep his stride unbroken. There was too much noise to hear anything but I knew something was there just behind me. You can sense it. Once I had the running rail there was still more than a furlong to go so I gave him one more crack just to make him aware that we had not finished. I was a bit hopeful by then unless something finished at a sprint and that's unlikely in the National after four and a half miles. I picked my whip up in my right hand, waved it rhythmically in encouragement and just gave him two more slaps down the neck to make sure he did not relax.

At the elbow Spartan Missile, finishing with ferocious zest, caught and passed Royal Mail in a matter of strides and had closed the gap on the leader to perhaps three lengths. Aldaniti's tongue was still hanging out in exhaustion but driven with strength and purpose, matching the indomitable spirit of his jockey and urged on by the encouragement of thousands of beseeching supporters, he responded resolutely to repel the fierce late thrust of Spartan Missile.

The gap, quite suddenly, was not shrinking any more and with a hundred yards to go it was clear to those who could bear to watch that Aldaniti and his remarkable rider were actually going to win. On they galloped to complete a glorious exhibition of soaring courage that, thanks to television, soon echoed around the world.

As Aldaniti galloped past the finishing post, his jockey waved his right hand exultantly high in the air—a spontaneous gesture of sheer, unbridled joy.

Chapter 19

JOSH GIFFORD, WHO had been unable to hold his binoculars steady throughout the race, was for once silent as his horse and jockey won the Grand National. Josh, who had never lost faith in Aldaniti and Bob Champion, stood speechless, almost numb, tears of emotion seeping down his face. Beside him his wife Althea and son Nick, the entire Embiricos family and Bob's girlfriend Jo were all overcome by the emotion of the occasion.

High up in the grandstand Carol and Jenny, the two girls who had nursed Bob through the darkest hours of his illness, clung to each other as floods of tears coursed down their cheeks. Carol had invested £3 on Aldaniti but never was a wager less important. Neither of the girls had brought race glasses and though they were well enough placed to see the fairytale finish their eyes were shut for most of the last, tense seconds of the drama.

Down at Lingfield in Surrey Bob's mother did not dare watch the race on television. She hid in the kitchen until her husband, Bob Champion senior, viewing on television in the next room, called out that Aldaniti was leading at the final fence. Phyllis Champion rushed into the room to see the finish, spotted Spartan Missile closing relentlessly on Aldaniti and dashed back at once to the safety of the kitchen sobbing unashamedly.

In Wiltshire Bob's sister Mary and her family, who had provided such solid and vital support throughout his illness, watched the race on television at a friend's house. Richard Hussey is a big, tough, practical man not usually given to emotion or sentiment, yet he trembled uncontrollably throughout the running of the 1981 Grand National. During the weeks before the race Mary had been having a recurring dream in which Aldaniti led going to the last fence, but she always woke up before the finish. Unable to sleep at all on the

200

eve of the National she was up at three in the morning washing and ironing, and was close to nervous exhaustion by the time the race began. Watching on television Mary dissolved into tears as early as the sixth fence, certain by then that her brother would win, and throughout the rest of that superb, unforgettable race she wept tears of joy with her two children beside her.

Patients and nursing staff gathered round the television in the Pinkham ward at the Royal Marsden Hospital in Sutton and shouted, roared and cheered Bob and Aldaniti on to victory in unison. Dr Jane Merrow, who listened to the race on the radio for the very good reason that she does not possess a television, says: "The atmosphere in the ward and indeed the entire hospital over the weekend was electric. Bob's success gave an enormous psychological boost to everyone there. It was such a fantastic achievement and the very best justification of what we put people through. Bob was the first person who had shown you can get back to complete fitness after the treatment and his win made the awful discomfort of the chemotherapy worthwhile."

No wonder Dr Merrow was delighted. She perhaps more than anyone else realized what a glorious advertisement Bob's victory had been for the dramatic breakthrough in the treatment of his illness. Until 1976 ninety per cent of all people suffering from his particular form of cancer died. The vital success of chemotherapy techniques had ensured that by April 1981 eighty per cent of patients not only survived but were able to recover completely.

At Liverpool Bob Champion and Aldaniti came back to one of the most emotional receptions ever witnessed at a sporting event. Thousands dashed headlong from the stands to greet them at the ancient wooden covered enclosure reserved for the winning team. Hundred of others charged out onto the course to applaud the heroes of the hour on their triumphant way back. Peter Double, the young lad who had looked after Aldaniti for three years, struggled through a mass of people to reach his horse. Bob, who was not blowing at all, leaned over and shouted, "*Did* you see him jump the Chair?"

"No," replied Peter. "I didn't see a thing throughout the race!"

Snowy Davis, fifty-five years in racing, had never known a

welcoming party like it. "I couldn't get anywhere near the horse's head. There was a wall of lunatics in front of me pulling and tugging at Aldaniti and a bloody great police horse treading on my heels. I'm lucky to have survived to tell the tale." Even so, extraordinarily fit and agile, Snowy eventually battled his way through to his rightful position beside Aldaniti.

John Thorne, forgetting his own disappointment at finishing second, rode over and clapped Bob generously on the back. "A marvellous result," John said later. "I was pleased with my horse and even more delighted for Bob. His win is the best story this century. Just the boost the country needs to cheer everyone up."

Soon Aldaniti and his smiling jockey came into sight flanked by the traditional escort of four massive mounted police horses. Althea Gifford somehow managed to move close enough to congratulate Bob and gain her reward when he leaned down to give her a warm kiss on the cheek. As horse and rider reached the winner's enclosure the waves of sustained applause reached a new crescendo that surpassed even the reception given to Red Rum after his historic third victory in the 1977 Grand National. Bob jumped down from Aldaniti's back and spoke briefly to Nick and Valda Embiricos and Josh Gifford.

Josh reminded me to weigh in. Quite right, too. He's a professional. I said he'd better come with me to make sure but he shook his head. They were all in floods of tears in there. Me? I didn't have time to cry. In the next ninety minutes I was pushed and shunted, shoved and battered, picked up and taken to a dozen different places. My feet didn't touch the ground and I didn't have a chance to speak to the boys in the weighing-room although I managed to organize two cases of champagne to be sent into them.

While the cheers continued Bob was escorted by two particularly beefy members of the Liverpool Constabulary to the scales where he removed his crash helmet and weighed in correctly at 10 stone 13 pounds. He sat on the scales, his saddle in one hand, brushed away the sweat from his pale, exultant face, delighted, astonished and just a little self-conscious in front of the television cameras. Moments later he was hustled out to the winners' enclosure again for the first of numerous interviews.

"What was second?" he asked David Coleman twice before he was given the answer.

After a brief interview by Coleman, Bob was taken to a small, shabby room filled with newspaper reporters, radio and television news men eager to question him. Bob's greatest moment of peril on Grand National day came at the start of the impromptu press conference as the stool he was offered collapsed under him. Not for the first time in the afternoon he demonstrated his excellent balance and remained on his feet as the stool, minus a leg, crashed to the ground. The story of his remarkable recovery from cancer had been well chronicled in the previous few days but Bob dealt patiently with an endless series of questions about his illness. Typically, he tried to divert attention from himself.

> Don't forget the trainer. What a great piece of training to bring Aldaniti back to win the National after three bad injuries and only one run in eighteen months.

Again Bob was pressed about his illness. Talking softly, picking his words carefully, he replied:

> I rode this race for all the patients in hospital. And all the people who look after them. My only wish is that my winning shows them that there is always hope, and all battles can be won. I just hope it will encourage others to face their illness with fresh spirit.

Bob gave numerous similar interviews until it was time for his second ride of the day on Homeson, trained by Josh Gifford, in a novice hurdle. Homeson, who started second favourite, flattered briefly on the final turn but faded badly and Bob was not hard on him when his chance was gone.

"I don't know why I bother to employ you," laughed Josh as his jockey came back to weigh in.

"That Gifford's a hard man," said Bob, who did not realize the trainer was joking. "I've just won the National and now I get a bollocking."

At last Bob and Jo were able to escape the attentions of the media. After a quick word with Carol and Jenny, they moved off to the car park, Bob clutching the sole remaining bottle of champagne from the two dozen he had bought for his fellow jockeys. On the way south he stopped at a service station to buy an evening newspaper.

"There you are, I'm not kidding myself. I did *win* the National!" he declared jubilantly as he looked at the headlines heralding his triumph only hours earlier. While he was at the service station there was time to ring his parents, sister and one or two close friends.

Later that night he stopped at the Westgate Hotel at Warwick for dinner as the guest of John Thorne and his family. While the rest of us ate and drank unstintingly the two men who had shared one of the most memorable finishes in the history of the Grand National were unable to enjoy the festivities fully. John Thorne, who had already devoured two small cakes at Liverpool, restricted himself to a small portion of whitebait and five figs. Bob chose a steak. Dinner finished just in time for everyone to watch the late-night showing of the race on BBC television. After it was over George Sloan, John Thorne's son-in-law, proposed a toast to two winners in the Grand National . . . Bob Champion and John Thorne.

Bob finally reached home just after two o'clock on Sunday morning. As he walked through the door the telephone was ringing with a call from Burly Cocks in America and the Ansafone was full of messages of congratulations. He managed a few hours' sleep before the telephone began ringing again at seven o'clock. It continued, unabated, until he left for Findon at midday to join the welcoming party for Aldaniti's homecoming. He imagined two or three hundred people might turn out in the cold, damp weather to see Aldaniti led out of his horsebox and was quite astonished at the sight of more than three thousand blocking the narrow village street.

Josh Gifford, who had been unable to watch the race objectively at the time, had since been studying it closely on his video recorder. As he poured endless glasses of champagne for his many guests he was full of praise for his horse and jockey. "Bob and Aldaniti went out there together and made the race their own. They joined together, as one, were united from the word go and put up a quite staggering performance. They gritted their teeth, refused to give in and just when I thought Royal Mail and Spartan Missile were coming to do us on the run-in they showed great guts to battle home together. Bob gave the horse the most brilliant ride and Aldaniti did his part perfectly."

In his supreme moment of triumph, Bob, unfailingly modest, insisted on giving all the credit to the horse who had carried him gloriously over four and a half miles and thirty of the most fearsome fences in the world.

Aldaniti is unbelievably tough. I always knew he would gallop until he dropped and I'm convinced that if, during the race, I had pointed him at a twenty-foot brick wall he would have gone straight through it. He was exhausted at the end but however tired he would have kept galloping for ten miles. *His* guts won the race. Nothing else.

I must admit I thought if I won the Grand National it would be one of the seven wonders of the world. It proves miracles do happen. Some people wrote us off as two old crocks together but I think we proved in the race we are not quite past it yet.

You can never fully accept that you are going to win the National, just as no-one really thinks they are going to collect on the football pools. You just hope and pray. I'm quite good at hoping. You shouldn't be in the job if you don't believe in certain things.

For me winning the National is like winning a gold medal at the Olympic Games or becoming a World Boxing Champion. It's a race I've always wanted to win so badly and I'm lucky to have done it. So many great jockeys have never had any luck at Liverpool. People like Jonjo O'Neill, Jeff King and Ron Barry. I didn't believe it had happened until we passed the post, or the lollypop stick as I call it. I still don't believe it some of the time. Well, did anyone really believe it?

Bob's victory on Aldaniti in the Grand National was the 393rd of his career and his 35th of the season.

That total pleased me no end because it equalled my score for the season before I was ill. That had always been my aim though at times it must have looked a bit ambitious. I'd like to go on riding for at least another year, maybe longer, until I don't enjoy it any more. Then my wish is to stay in racing in some capacity. I've always been keen to train horses one day but that's such an expensive business.

Bob's Liverpool triumph gained him several more awards including a television video recorder and yet more champagne. He won the video recorder, complete with film of the 1981 Grand National, for the most outstanding riding performance in the race. The man behind the award was Ted Dexter, the former England cricket captain who now runs his own public relations business. He introduced the award in 1978 on the basis that riding in the Grand National is not simply about winning but also taking on a terrifying ordeal. I imagine the two judges, Lord Oaksey and Richard Pitman, did not have to waste too much time on debate before choosing Bob Champion. Ted Dexter Associates also presented a cheque for £250 to the Injured Jockeys Fund. Bob won a Jeroboam of Mumm champagne too, the equivalent of four bottles, from the *Observer* newspaper as their Sports Personality of the week. Bookmakers refused to name the odds about Bob being voted Amoco Jockey of the Month for the third time in five months—which he duly was.

Bob was inundated with dozens of requests for personal appearances at functions varying from a Royal picnic to opening a pigeon fanciers fete in Yorkshire. He was particularly pleased to be invited as guest of honour to two boxing dinners in the West End of London to raise funds for the Royal Marsden Hospital in Sutton. Dennis Floyd, field officer in the UK and Overseas for the Cancer Research Campaign, lost no time in arranging for Aldaniti and his jockey to be the star attraction at the sponsored picnic in Windsor Great Park on 4th July. Both the Queen and the Queen Mother were due to attend this major fund-raising event which was expected to attract half a million people, and Bob promised to fly back from his working holiday in America to be there.

Dennis Floyd was extravagant in his praise of Bob Champion. "Bob's victory in the Grand National is the greatest thing that has happened in the fifty-year history of the campaign. His fantastic achievement shows that modern techniques have helped to cure several types of cancer and he has given the most enormous inspiration and hope to the younger people who have cancer. His indomitable spirit and courage have proved that people *can* survive this terrible illness. I think he is the most marvellous chap."

The 1981 Grand National, sponsored by the *Sun* newspaper, was seen around the world, either live or recorded, by a massive audience estimated at seven hundred and fifty million people. The BBC employed no fewer than twenty cameras for their superb, comprehensive coverage that was watched in Great Britain alone by eighteen million viewers. On Sunday the race was broadcast coast to coast in America by NBC.

Anyone watching on television in the comfort of their own home would have had a much better view than the huge crowd of 67,000 packed tight in the racecourse's ancient grandstands and enclosures. Liverpool is such an enormous racecourse and the runners go so far away from the stands that it is quite impossible to follow the race with any accuracy. However unsatisfactory the viewing arrangements, though, there can be no better argument for the continuation of the Grand National than its result in 1981 which proved universally popular. There were twelve finishers, and of those who did not complete the course none of the horses or jockeys suffered anything more than a few scratches. Aldaniti devoured his evening meal with his usual enthusiasm and returned to Findon sound and in excellent spirits. He was retired for the season but may be given the chance to return to Aintree next year to attempt a second famous victory.

Despite massive favourable publicity, a huge attendance and a vast television audience round the world, the Grand National's future seemed in serious doubt in the weeks after the 1981 race. Ladbrokes' contract to run the meeting was due to expire in 1982 and several offers by them to purchase the course from the owner Bill Davies had been sharply rejected. Since 1945 there had been a series of "last" Nationals. The course had changed hands several times but various schemes to safeguard the future of the race had failed. The ugly shadow of property development remained ever present.

Each year, for one all too brief golden hour, the Grand National offers drama and optimism, pathos and tragedy, courage and endurance. The race is part of the nation's heritage, a unique, unrivalled event cherished in Great Britain and admired throughout the rest of the world. Whatever the cost, whatever the problem, it must not be allowed to die.

In the days after the 1981 Grand National Bob Champion was overwhelmed by the sheer volume of telegrams, messages, letters, drawings and poems he received. Some one thousand arrived within a week of the race. First among them was a telegram from Josh Gifford and Aldaniti saying, "Congratulations after a brave fight."

The Queen Mother's private secretary Sir Martin Gilliat wrote. "I am delighted to convey to you Queen Elizabeth, The Queen Mother's warmest congratulations on your wonderful victory. Your success brought to Her Majesty enormous pleasure as it undoubtedly did to millions in all parts of the world."

A letter arrived from Prince Charles, at the time in the middle of a hectic official visit to New Zealand and Australia. The Prince, whose own brief attempts as a steeplechase jockey in the previous months had left no-one in doubt about his courage or commitment to the sport, sent a warm message of congratulations in his own hand: "I simply *had* to write a short letter of admiration following your wonderful win in the Grand National. It really was the best possible news after your illness and the troubles with Aldaniti and I am so glad that fate has been so generous to you at last. With my very best wishes and renewed congratulations. Charles."

Dr Jane Merrow sent a telegram saying, "Congratulations on winning the race and the fight. We are all delighted." Another doctor from Bob's hospital wrote: "I felt I simply had to congratulate you on a wonderful personal achievement which boosted us all tremendously. I am sure you realize we are all extremely proud of you."

Kybo's owners Isidore and Blanche Kerman said: "We were thrilled at seeing you win the Grand National on television. We are so happy for you." Blanche Kerman sent a separate note which read: "Aldaniti is a good horse but without you Bob he could not have won because you nursed him all the way over the jumps."

One telegram, from Pat Betts, contained a tentative booking for

Bob in the 1984 Grand National: "Congratulations on a fantastic achievement. You are a great credit to a wonderful sport. PS Can I book you now for Abbey Brig in the 1984 Grand National?" Eleven days later at Ascot, Abbey Brig was to be Bob's first winner since the National.

Still the messages continued to pour in, many of them from people Bob did not know who were so moved by his success and quiet dignity afterwards that they felt they just had to write to him.

Clive and Leslie Bailey, old friends from Bob's days with Toby Balding, wrote: "Words cannot express our joy. Fantastic. God bless you."

Nick and Frisky Nutting sent a telegram saying, "Always thought you were Champion. You have proved us right."

A former girlfriend summed up the prevailing mood of emotion: "Bob with lots of cheers and floods of tears."

Diane Oughton, widow of Josh Gifford's friend Alan Oughton, who died of cancer, wrote simply, "Bob you are the greatest."

There was a telegram, too, from the Park Street Clinic, still in operation despite the tragic death of Alun Thomas.

Two bank managers from Wootton Bassett added their own congratulations. One commented, "Might I explain that several members of my staff here are richer than they were on Friday night?" His rival from another bank in the same town said brightly, "Let me know in advance if you are going to do it again."

More telegrams and letters were delivered. Colm and Lizzie Farren said briefly and accurately, "You wrote the best chapter of all today."

A woman from Norfolk wrote: "Thank you for winning the Grand National. Thank you from someone who spends much of her time nursing cancer patients. Your achievement on Saturday will give cancer sufferers all over the world terrific encouragement and a great deal of hope. Your courage and fortitude will be a terrific boost for people at this present time undergoing depressive chemotherapy and cancer operations."

An old girlfriend from America sent a long, emotional letter saying, "Your courage, determination and skill has carried you to the threshold of being a legend. You will journey beyond immortality around the world and with the respect, admiration and love of those whose lives you've touched. The thrill of life itself and the epitome of steeplechasing met when you crossed the finish line on Aldaniti."

There was a telegram and a warm letter from Bob's most loyal fan, Eunice Brooker from Brighton. Since 1976 Eunice had been knitting him three or four sweaters each year and had been a regular correspondent during his illness.

Another of his doctors from the Royal Marsden Hospital wrote, "Needless to say I was absolutely delighted by your triumph on Saturday. Your example will be a great one for many other patients with cancer. It has provided the patients and staff of this hospital with a great emotional boost."

Bob Champion, the man in receipt of such a continuous stream of praise, admiration and at times adulation, was curiously unimpressed by his own performance in winning the Grand National. While he was in hospital his impossible dream that he would triumph in the National on Aldaniti had developed into an obsession. He alone, through months of anguish, torment and doubt, had believed he would recover sufficiently to ride again.

All right. I'm pleased I've won the race every jockey wants to win more than any other. It's been the biggest ambition of my life and I've achieved it. But my part was the easy bit. Any competent professional would have won on Aldaniti. I was fortunate to be on the right horse on the right day.

Totally unassuming, Bob insists quite seriously:

I haven't done anything really because I only sat on the horse for ten minutes or so. All the work has been done by Josh and his lads, the owners and their staff who got Aldaniti ready each time to send back into training. They had the patience, good sense and faith in the horse to give him the necessary amount of time on the three occasions they nursed him back to health. As for my part, as I've said before, most important of all I just hope my victory will give other patients who have had the disease a little bit of hope.

It's strange really. When I was so ill in hospital many people

210

told me I was mad even to consider risking my neck by riding again when I recovered, but they don't understand me. You see I still enjoy racing. It's my life. I like the risk part of it. I always have done. If I'd been stopped from riding again I'd have tried rally driving, scrambling or even motor racing. anything with an element of danger.

People make a lot of fuss about our so-called bravery and courage. All this talk about heroics is nonsense. We all know the risks and accept them. In our game you expect bumps and bruises. There's nothing to match the thrill of riding good horses at speed over fences. *Nothing*. I don't see that courage has anything to do with it. It's simply a job we all enjoy doing.

For the last words on this extraordinary man, consider the definition of the word "champion" in *Chambers Twentieth Century Dictionary:*

One who fights in single combat for himself or for another: one who defends a cause: a successful combatant: in sports, one who has excelled all others: a hero.

Index

Index

*denotes the name of a horse

215

Harry Cole

POLICEMAN'S PROGRESS

Being one of four policemen coping with the drunken, sex-mad, middle-aged, pear-shaped Clara, or sitting out a night with the neighbourhood ghost, or calming wayward Rosie, the local prostitute, who'd had her 'Bristols' bitten, must have been a lot more fun than digging out the late and seventy-year-old Elsie Morton, rotting in bed after not being seen for some weeks, dealing with violence, or bearing the news of fatal accidents to bereaved families.

PC Harry Cole, now nearly thirty years on the Southwark force, has done it all and there's consequently many a tale to tell. He produces his account of life on the beat with a combination of good humour and honesty that makes *Policeman's Progress* a rich mixture of riotous and serious reading. Harry Cole's loyalty to the force, but also his obvious sympathy for all reasonable human eccentricities, make one feel that he would be a good man to have around when there's trouble.

Helen Forrester

TWOPENCE TO CROSS THE MERSEY

Helen Forrester tells the sad but never sentimental story of her childhood years, during which her family fell from genteel poverty to total destitution. In the depth of the Depression, mistakenly believing that work would be easier to find, they moved from the South of England to the slums of Liverpool. Here Helen Forrester, the eldest of seven children, experienced the worst degradations that being poor can bring. She writes about them without self-pity but rather with a rich sense of humour which makes her account of these grim days before the Welfare State funny as well as painful.

'The clarity with which utter privation is here recorded is of a rare kind' – Gillian Reynolds, *Guardian*

'. . . records, with remarkable steadiness and freedom from self-pity, the story of a childhood that – even if it was all forty years ago – most people would have set down in rage and despair' – Edward Blishen, *Books and Bookmen*

'. . . her restraint and humour in describing this stark history make it all the more moving' – *Daily Telegraph*

John Barnes

EVA PERON

Beautiful, brave, unscrupulous, Eva Perón rose from grinding poverty to become the glittering, hypnotically powerful First Lady of Argentina. To the millions of Argentina's poor, 'the shirtless ones', she was the saint who built them hospitals and homes, gave them food and clothes and money. They called her Santa Evita, Our Lady of Hope. To her enemies, and she had plenty, she was a monstrous dictator whose Social Aid charity was the world's most gigantic protection racket-cum-slush fund.

John Barnes explores the astonishing paradox of this socialite, feminist and champion of the poor who attacked the rich yet made herself a multi-millionairess. Even in death she haunts Argentina. Her embalmed body, stolen after she died in 1952, was 'discovered' twenty years later and finally buried in 1976. Yet her charisma still lives on. In Argentina today she is as loved and as hated as ever.

Fontana Paperbacks: Non-fiction

Fontana is a leading paperback publisher of non-fiction, both popular and academic. Below are some recent titles.

- ☐ MARY ELLEN'S HELP YOURSELF DIET PLAN £1.50
- ☐ POLICEMAN'S PATROL Harry Cole £1.50
- ☐ MACROECONOMICS Wynne Godley & Francis Cripps £3.95
- ☐ POEMS AND SONGS OF ROBERT BURNS £2.95
- ☐ LAND OF THE SCOTS: A SHORT HISTORY Caroline Bingham £1.95
- ☐ BY THE WATERS OF LIVERPOOL Helen Forrester £1.95
- ☐ WHAT LANDS ARE THESE? Dorothy Hammond Innes £1.75
- ☐ HITCH-HIKER'S GUIDE TO EUROPE Ken Welsh £2.95
- ☐ UNDERSTANDING AND PRODUCING SPEECH T. Roeper & E. Matthei £2.95
- ☐ HOME-MADE PRESERVES Jill Nice £3.50
- ☐ NEW INDIAN COOKERY Meera Taneja £2.95
- ☐ GREEK FOOD Rena Salaman £2.95
- ☐ ENGLAND AND ITS RULERS Michael Clanchy £3.50
- ☐ EUROPE TRANSFORMED Norman Stone £3.50
- ☐ JUNG: SELECTED WRITINGS ed. Anthony Storr £3.95
- ☐ THE HELEN SMITH STORY Paul Foot £2.50
- ☐ WILL THERE REALLY BE A MORNING? Frances Farmer £1.95
- ☐ BARTHES Jonathan Culler £1.75
- ☐ BETTER PROGRAMMING FOR YOUR SPECTRUM AND ZX81 Robert Speel £2.95
- ☐ MARX: THE FIRST HUNDRED YEARS ed. David McLellan £3.95

You can buy Fontana paperbacks at your local bookshop or newsagent. Or you can order them from Fontana Paperbacks, Cash Sales Department, Box 29, Douglas, Isle of Man. Please send a cheque, postal or money order (not currency) worth the purchase price plus 10p per book (or 12p per book if outside the UK).

NAME (Block letters) _____

ADDRESS _____

_____